Navigating Borderline Personality Disorder

*Strategies and Insights to Reduce Conflict,
Set Healthy Boundaries and Balance
Compassion with Self-Care*

Freeman Publishing

eBook ISBN 978-1-963333-08-4
Paperback ISBN 978-1-963333-09-1
Hardback ISBN 978-1-963333-03-9

Table of Contents

Introduction   7

1. UNDERSTANDING BORDERLINE
   PERSONALITY TRAITS   17
   What is Borderline Personality Disorder?   17
   Why Learn About Borderline Personality Disorder?   19
   The Diagnostic Process   20
   Borderline Personality Disorder Biology and Psychology   21
   Myth-Busting Borderline Personality Disorder   26
   Internalizing Your Knowledge   30
   Key Takeaways   30

2. AN EMOTIONAL ROLLERCOASTER: HIGHS
   AND LOWS OF BORDERLINE PERSONALITY
   DISORDER RELATIONSHIPS   33
   The Borderline Personality Disorder Relationship Cycle   33
   *What to Expect: How Borderline Personality Disorder
   Affects Relationships*   37
   Effects of Borderline Personality Disorder on Families   39
   There Are Also Positives!   40
   *Cultivating Positive Borderline Personality Disorder
   Relationships*   42
   Interactive Element   42
   Key Takeaways   43

3. EFFECTIVE COMMUNICATION STRATEGIES   45
   Validating Feelings   45
   Reducing Borderline Rage   49
   Tips for Managing Borderline Personality Disorder Anger   51
   For Individuals with BPD   51
   Trying to Fix Things   58
   Interactive Element: Dealing With Conflict   59
   Key Takeaways   59

4. SETTING BOUNDARIES WITHOUT
BUILDING WALLS   63
The Importance of Setting Healthy Boundaries   63
Types of Boundaries   66
Setting and Maintaining Clear Boundaries   67
*Boundaries and Emotional Detachment: What's the
Difference?*   68
Guilt-Free Boundary Setting   69
Interactive Element: Taking Action   71
Key Takeaways   72

5. COMPASSION VERSUS CODEPENDENCY—
FINDING THE BALANCE   77
What is Codependency?   77
*The Link Between Borderline Personality Disorder and
Codependency*   78
Differentiating Between Compassion and Codependency   79
Signs of Codependency   80
How to Stop Being Codependent   80
Support Versus Enabling   83
Practicing Mindfulness   86
Interactive Element: Becoming Your Own Person   88
Key Takeaways   88

6. DEALING WITH THE IMPACT OF BPD ON
YOUR MENTAL HEALTH   91
Recognizing Signs of Trauma   91
The Importance of Self-Care   93
10 Self-Care Ideas to Try   94
Using Breathing Techniques   96
Staying Healthy   100
Interactive Element: Prioritizing Yourself   104
Key Takeaways   105

7. THERAPEUTIC APPROACHES AND THEIR
EFFICACY   107
Treatment Options for Borderline Personality Disorder   107
*Encouraging Therapy for Individuals with Borderline
Personality Disorder*   111
Success Stories   115

Interactive Element: Choosing the Right Treatment   117
Key Takeaways   117

8. SEEKING SUPPORT FROM GROUPS TO
   PROFESSIONALS   119
   The Benefits of Support Groups   119
   Seeking Support for Yourself   121
   Talking to Others   124
   Resources for Caregivers   125
   Interactive Element: Getting Much-Needed Support   127
   Key Takeaways   128

9. NAVIGATING BREAKUPS AND LETTING GO   131
   Until Borderline Personality Disorder, Do Us Part   131
   Handling Breakups with Care and Sensitivity   134
   Moving On and Letting Go   136
   Case Studies   138
   Interactive Element: Putting Yourself First   142
   Key Takeaways   142

Conclusion   145
References   149

Introduction

From the moment you first laid eyes on each other, you just knew you had to be together. They're attractive, friendly, funny, and sexy. You like the same things, and the chemistry between you is electric. Soon after meeting, they bombard you with romantic texts. They tell you that you're the best thing that ever happened to them. Whatever you're into, they embrace it. They will do crossword puzzels, run marathons, or visit art galleries just because you like to. You're flattered. When your relationship becomes physical—which happens quickly—the sex is amazing. No relationship has ever been quite like this. You've met your soulmate. Within weeks, you're living together, or perhaps you're planning your wedding. This is the best time of your life.

Until the bubble bursts. On your honeymoon you're accused of cheating when you're polite to other guests. They give you the silent treatment. You don't know what you've done, and they won't tell you. Mystified, you presume—incorrectly—that this was just a blip. You move into your new home. You soon find out that they quit their job before the wedding without telling you; they're a big spender; they drink more alcohol than you realized; they lie needlessly; they have no friends; they fly into rages at the slightest provocation; and they have precipitous mood swings. The worst of it is that they're just getting started.

When the relationship works, you feel as though you've inherited all the stars in the sky. Just days or even hours later, you're like a tramp, searching through the trash for scraps of their affection. Often, their feelings for you appear to be as ephemeral as mist, turning you into an emotional skeleton watching the clouds cover the moon.

You meet your new best friend at a party. She's quirky and funny. You seem to share the same interests, so you swap phone numbers. You go out for pizza and have a great time. Before you know it, she's bombarding you with texts and invitations. She gets upset if you don't respond to her texts or return her phone calls promptly or when you can't see her because you have other commitments. After a while, she belittles you. She shouts at you in public and swears at you on the phone. She is very apologetic afterward, but you wonder if you need a friend like this. You try to back off, but she's not having it.

These normal, everyday relationships rapidly become intense, demanding, and extreme. You receive contradictory texts at random times during the day. This person is oddly needy and loves picking explosive, pointless arguments. The lying soon reaches pathological levels.

Suddenly, you're the problem. You don't care about them; you neglected them when you visited a sick relative in the hospital; their ex was much kinder; they loathe the activities you enjoy. They're contradictory, rapidly moving from being clinging vines to becoming vicious ice queens. Arguments never get resolved. They have no boundaries. You're embarrassed in public and insulted or even assaulted in private. They will literally scream to get your attention. An hour later, they're telling you to go away, or they are stonewalling you. They threaten to leave, only to come back and beg forgiveness in an endless cycle.

You're riding an emotional rollercoaster blindfolded. There are no beacons on this dark, stormy sea your relationship or friendship has become. You care for them, but you tiptoe around them. You're frightened of who they are, and you don't recognize who you're becoming.

Eventually, you might discover the deeply buried hurt at the heart of their bizarre behavior—childhood abandonment, neglect, or abuse. You know you can leave, but you don't. You peer beyond the wreckage to the wonderful person hiding beneath the pain. In their more lucid moments, you know they see the good in you, but they're terrified that it will somehow evaporate. You want the relationship to work if only you can get beyond their bizarre behavior.

You might have a daughter who is disruptive. She won't listen to anyone or do anything she's asked to do. Your home life is a nightmare of fights and arguments. She drinks excessively and shouts at everyone, saying she hates them. The other siblings ignore her. Your husband works longer hours. You don't feel you have anyone to turn to. She talks about having suicidal thoughts. You dismiss it, thinking she's just acting out. One day, you walk into her room and find her cut to ribbons, with blood all over the floor. The trauma lives on in your mind. You realize your daughter is deeply disturbed. You've done nothing wrong, but you can't sleep at night because of the terror and the guilt.

These strange behaviors are all symptoms of borderline personality disorder (BPD). Sometimes, it's diagnosed, but often, it's not. While some sufferers make heroic efforts to resolve their problems, others will hide them and would rather bleed or run off with a lover their partner never knew existed—or tear family or friendships apart—then let anyone see their angst.

Profiling Borderline Personality Disorder

Borderline Personality Disorder (BPD) is a mental condition where sufferers find it difficult to temper their emotional responses to people and situations. They feel emotions intensely and may take a long time to wind down after a triggering event.

BPD affects only 1.6% of the adult population in the United States, which equates to over four million people. That might be an underestimate, however—some sources put it as high as 5.9%. Around three-quarters of those living with BPD are female. Males may incorrectly be diagnosed with Post-Traumatic Stress Disorder (PTSD) or depression (ADAMHS, 2006). The condition usually manifests when people are in their late teens or early twenties. Family history, genetics, and socioeconomic factors all play a role.

Signs of BPD may include (ADAMHS, 2006):

- poor self-image
- impulsiveness
- desperation to avoid actual or perceived abandonment by friends, family, and romantic partners
- stormy relationships
- intense emotional responses to stressful events and situations
- low moods, irritability, anxiety, or severe depression

- feelings of emptiness or boredom
- intense, inappropriate anger followed by guilt and shame
- feelings of disconnection
- paranoia triggered by stress, sometimes manifesting as psychotic episodes
- self-harm

Relating to People Living with Personality Disorder

Having a relationship with someone diagnosed with BPD presents its own set of difficulties that can be excruciating to deal with. They will foist the blame for deficiencies in their relationships on their partners, parents, siblings, and friends, although their behavior is not the result of anything anyone else might have said or done. They have little control over their BPD behaviors—and neither do those with whom they interact.

Having someone with BPD in your life means that it's important to understand some of the ways in which the condition manifests. This isn't a magic book, but it will help you gain perspective and avoid some of the emotional and psychological damage these relationships can inflict on unsuspecting partners, spouses, family members, and friends.

The core belief that underpins BPD is the terror of being abandoned. Although these beliefs don't always have apparent triggers, very often, it's a response to childhood sexual abuse. It might seem counterintuitive, but such people are often sexually impulsive and even promiscuous, so romantic relationships rapidly become physical. Sufferers might have multiple sexual partners who don't always know about one another and move back and forth between them.

Individuals with BPD may become unusually clingy, inappropriately demanding, and jealous, convinced despite the evidence that their loved ones will leave or betray them. An uncle might notice that his nephew acts paranoid in social situations, convinced that others are talking about him behind his back. There may be no history of abuse, yet a daughter might develop an inexplicable eating disorder or threaten to murder her father during an argument.

People with BPD fear real intimacy—they don't want to get too close to someone who might leave them. This expresses itself as severe moodiness. Unfortunately, these unchecked behaviors destabilize their relationships.

Lying is another common BPD trait, which further undermines the trust inherent in a close relationship. Many people with BPD are chronic liars and don't seem to realize the damage lying may do, much less feel remorseful about spinning a host of fictional narratives.

It can be frightening and disconcerting to be close to someone who suffers from BPD. Their erratic, bizarre, and even abusive behaviors take a tremendous toll on the mental and psychological health of those around them. There is a brief respite, and even positive experiences can quickly spiral into drama. As around half of the people with BPD are not regularly employed, their partners and family members have the added burden of providing for them financially and materially. All this can be overwhelming and exhausting.

Those who have BPD develop an intense, exclusive attachment to their romantic partners, spouses, or friends, who then need to fulfill all their material, emotional, and spiritual needs. Relationships become unbalanced. It becomes difficult for those involved to flourish and reach their own potential. Those closest to the individual risk becoming islands—marooned on the shores of their whims, needs, and desires, with no one to share the burden.

Friendships struggle, with the individual sharing little of themselves and often demanding far more than the other person can reasonably be expected to give. Friendships may be stormy, alternating between adoration and angry accusations. Ignore their texts at your peril. Those with BPD who experience severe symptoms may have few close friends. This may change with treatment, however, and those who have learned to confront their demons actually make wonderful, good, and loyal friends.

How This Book May Help You

If someone close to you has BPD, you will know how paradoxical it can feel. You care about them, and you're concerned about their welfare despite ongoing drama and constant disruptions. You see beyond the facade to the inability to cope with inordinately painful life experiences. You would like nothing better than to see them healed and whole and to have a rich and fulfilling relationship with the person they might be.

Although you may feel marooned and powerless, you are not alone. There are several famous people who clawed their way back from BPD to experience rich, rewarding relationships with people who stood by them through their best times and their worst. Following diagnosis and treatment, some have used their struggles to help others emerge victorious.

Former NFL running back, Heisman Trophy winner, and actor Ricky Williams revealed that he'd been diagnosed with several issues, including BPD, and has been raising awareness of mental health issues across cultures and races. Brandon Marshall, another former football great, has been treated for BPD and is working to reduce the stigma around mental health. Actress Madison Bailey struggles with BPD and supports others in seeking help. Comedian Pete Davidson is also diagnosed with BPD and encourages those with the diagnosis to work toward living normal, happier lives.

Dr. Marsha Linehan is a psychologist whose story shows that being diagnosed with BPD can be a life-changing experience—in a good way. Dr. Linehan was incorrectly diagnosed with schizophrenia as a teen after experiencing debilitating headaches, suicidal tendencies, and a propensity for self-harm. Psychotic medications and therapies left her with amnesia and reduced brain function at 17. One year later, she self-diagnosed with BPD. She spent years studying psychology, working as a lecturer and professor, and volunteering at the 988 Lifeline (Better Help Editorial Team, 2023).

Her award-winning research into suicidal tendencies culminated in the creation of a form of cognitive-behavioral therapy called Dialectical Behavioral Therapy (DBT). This therapy focuses on mindfulness, improved interpersonal effectiveness, emotional control, and stress tolerance. Her work stemmed from the belief that suicide is a response to extreme emotional pain. In the late 1960s, she was recovering from a psychiatric episode when she enrolled at Loyola, spending time in the organization's chapel. While praying, she finally realized that she was acceptable, even with all her faults and difficult emotions, and stopped self-harming. Radical acceptance lies at the heart of DBT (Better Help Editorial Team, 2023).

Real love comes from communication and understanding. You might struggle to bridge the gap between your loved one's perception of the world and reality. You want them to know how much you care while still preserving your sense of self.

How do you do this authentically without triggering your loved one's deep-seated insecurities and setting them off? How do you create and enforce boundaries in your relationship without constantly having to sacrifice your own needs? You are as much a victim of their pain as they are—and they may make you feel as though all their problems are your fault. This can be unsettling. Although you know this cannot logically be the case, you somehow feel responsible.

While there is ultimately hope for people with BPD, you might wonder how much longer you can hang on as you wait for them to realize that they themselves need to take the first steps toward improving their own mental health. Their all-consuming needs might make you feel guilty about your own need to express yourself, be yourself, and take time out. The trouble is that a person with BPD knows this and might exploit your feelings. How do you find the balance between their needs and yours?

This book will help you both understand and manage your loved one's BPD and its effects while still keeping your sense of self. It will help you end the endless guilt trips and evolve from being codependent to being a person in your own right. In this book, you'll find out how to navigate the complexities of caring about someone who has BPD and develop effective strategies for communicating more effectively while maintaining your own well-being.

In this book, you'll discover self-help techniques that will enable you to become objective about your relationship and their dysfunctionality. You'll learn how to love individuals with BPD and communicate with them without getting drawn into whatever drama is dominating the day. You'll find out how to do reality checks to protect yourself from behaviors like gaslighting, guilt-tripping, lying, circular arguments, and endless hurt and fear.

After reading this book, you can finally get off the emotional rollercoaster by following its guidelines through the toxic BPD maze so that you can offer effective help and support for your loved one while loving yourself and staying strong.

Chapter 1

Understanding Borderline Personality Traits

 "Your struggles do not define you, but they can refine you."

— Reyna I. Aburto

Maintaining a relationship with someone suffering from BPD can be very challenging, so it's helpful to understand the reasons for their behavior. In this chapter, you'll discover the characteristics of BPD, the diagnostic process, the reasons it evolves, and some myths that surround the condition.

What is Borderline Personality Disorder?

BPD is a personality disorder or mental illness that makes it difficult to manage emotions. BPD is also referred to by different names, including Emotionally Unstable Personality Disorder (EUPD), Emotional Intensity Disorder (EID), and Borderline Pattern Personality Disorder (BPPD) (Mind, 2022).

Signs and Symptoms

One of the chief characteristics of BPD is violent swings from one end of the emotional spectrum to the other. Intense and unpredictable moodiness may be difficult to deal with. This can have a significant impact on your relationship with a person with BPD. They may be volatile, with their values and interests changing suddenly. They see everything in black-and-white and rarely acknowledge the shades of gray in between. The impulsiveness and recklessness typical of BPD may give those close to them anxious moments. Other indicators of BPD include:

- fear of being abandoned
- feeling disconnected from reality or other people
- a history of intense, unstable relationships and friendships
- a distorted sense of self and poor self-image
- suicidal threats and self-harming behaviors like cutting
- inconsistent, variable, and exaggerated moods
- difficulty controlling anger, which is often intense and inappropriate
- feelings of emptiness
- becoming paranoid or disassociating when extremely stressed
- impulsive, often hazardous behaviors—unsafe sex, reckless driving, substance misuse, spending sprees, and binge eating or drinking (National Institute of Mental Health, 2023)

Not everyone who has BPD will display all these symptoms; the severity and duration vary from one person to another. Many people with BPD self-harm and may be suicidal.

Why Learn About Borderline Personality Disorder?

BPD is a surprisingly complex condition. While receiving a diagnosis can clarify your situation, it might also require you to take a step back and see how you and your loved one with BPD can work together to manage the emotional challenges BPD creates. Therefore, it's crucial that those whose friends, coworkers, or loved ones suffer from BPD learn as much as possible about the condition, how it manifests, and how to help reduce negative impacts.

Being informed can prepare you mentally and emotionally for the storms that accompany this condition. Empathize with your loved one, showing that you can appreciate what they are going through. You know their potential, and it can frustrate them that their diagnosis stymies their personal development. There are many ways to show support.

- Listen and acknowledge the person's feelings, even if they seem irrational. Many people with BPD experience tremendous guilt about their emotional outbursts and will be very relieved if you validate their emotions. Put yourself in their shoes and show understanding without judgment. This will help you respond with compassion and be supportive, especially when things get difficult. This can reduce their emotional distress and improve your connection.
- Be patient. This is easier said than done, as you might feel that your patience is exhausted, especially if you have been dealing with their behavior for some time.
- Avoid arguing. Wait until you can talk things over calmly. Don't climb onto their emotional rollercoaster. Their feelings may be overwhelming, so it will help to

diffuse the situation if you stay calm and respond consistently. You aren't a machine, so if you feel angry or upset, take time away. Do something you enjoy or go for a walk.

- People with BPD rarely see their own positive traits. Reminding them of these can help them feel loved, supported, and reassured. When they are calm and rational, talk to them and find out what you can do for them when their emotions become overwhelming.
- Find out what triggers them so you can be prepared and avoid situations that make them uncomfortable or reinforce their terrors of being abandoned, rejected, or alone. Do activities they enjoy. You can either suggest or simply start doing something, letting them know you would be happy for them to join you.

It's essential that you don't neglect your own needs. It can be demanding and stressful to look after someone with this condition, so elicit the help of other family members and friends and give yourself time out. The person with BPD will value your efforts and those of people in your circle to spend time with them and show them you care.

The Diagnostic Process

Only a licensed health professional may diagnose BPD in the United States. The diagnosis is based on a psychiatric interview and medical examination. Screenings can be done by psychologists, therapists, or clinical social workers. The assessment usually includes:

- a detailed interview and assessment of the patient's present symptoms and previous life history
- a review of the patient's medical history, as well as that of their family
- a medical exam to rule out other causes of symptoms (Krouse, 2023)

There are assessment tools designed specifically to diagnose BPD. At least five of the emotional difficulties mentioned previously need to be present (Krouse, 2023). While there are no laboratory tests required, additional tests might be conducted to rule out other causes of a person's symptoms.

Self-diagnosis is not typical. Many people occasionally experience symptoms of BPD but don't fit all the diagnostic criteria. This is further complicated by comorbidities, such as eating disorders or other conditions that sometimes manifest with BPD. The most prevalent are histrionic and narcissistic personality disorders. Around 60.5% of people with BPD have a linked anxiety disorder, while over 30% present with impulse control and substance abuse (Migala, 2022). Because symptoms often overlap, BPD can frequently be misdiagnosed.

Another reason for diagnostic delays is that BPD is difficult to treat, and patients might be stigmatized.

Borderline Personality Disorder Biology and Psychology

An increased understanding of brain chemistry is revealing the biological causes of BPD. The parts of the brain governing emotion and rational thought include the amygdala and the prefrontal cortex (PFC). The amygdala is part of the limbic system, which comprises the hippocampus, thalamus, hypothalamus, basal ganglia, and cingulate gyrus. These are found deep inside the brain and are where emotions are generated. The PFC is behind the forehead. It controls the brain's executive functions—regulating conflicting thoughts, differentiating between right and wrong, and enabling self-control. The PFC also regulates the amygdala and limbic system.

To explain this, consider this example: you're at a family reunion when your cousin trips and spills a glass of red wine on your favorite jacket. Your immediate impulse might be to shout at him, but doing so would cause an unpleasant scene. You decide to fetch another jacket from your vehicle and speak to him later. This is your PFC regulating your spontaneous emotional reaction. If your PFC was undeveloped or malfunctioning, you may have shouted impulsively at your cousin, potentially ruining the joyous atmosphere.

Studies have revealed that both the PFC and limbic system are underdeveloped in people with BPD, which makes them more impulsive (Collins, 2023). To compensate for this, the amygdala becomes hyperactive, which results in emotional reactions. Because emotional responses are heightened, the behavior of someone with BPD appears more extreme. The hyperactive, unregulated limbic system and amygdala create the overwhelming emotional experiences typical of BPD.

The amygdala also generates memories. Most of us learn from our negative experiences and avoid repeating our mistakes. When someone has BPD, negative emotional experiences replay in their heads, so they continuously re-experience them long after the actual events are over.

Borderline Personality Disorder and Neurotransmitters

Neurotransmitters are chemicals that transmit messages or signals from one nerve cell to the next and to other cells in the body. These signals travel rapidly through the body. Three different types of neurotransmitters have been studied regarding BPD:

- The body releases opiates to dull pain when injuries occur. Your brain makes its own versions of opioids, called endogenous opioids. Studies show that people with BPD who self-harm have lower levels of opiates in their bodies. Opiates lift one's mood, and at least some self-harming people with BPD may feel better. In an odd paradox, self-harmers experience mild physical pain like headaches, back pain, or abdominal pain more regularly than other people.
- Serotonin regulates sleep and mood while enabling learning. Individuals with BPD are typically deficient in serotonin, which aggravates aggressive and impulsive behavior.
- Cortisol is a stress hormone that initiates the flight-or-flight stress response, breaking down carbohydrates and proteins to increase the supply of oxygen and sugars to the brain, heart, and muscles. When cortisol levels remain high for long periods, this can cause high blood pressure, weight gain, bone-thinning, and immune system suppression. People with BPD frequently have high cortisol levels, potentially affecting the memory centers in the brain's hippocampus. This can generate suicidal thoughts (Collins, 2023).

The Role of Genetics

You share around 50% of your genes with close relatives like your parents, siblings, and children. If any of them have BPD, your chances of developing this condition are five times greater than if they didn't. Research into the prevalence of BPD in families has confirmed that the chances of developing the condition increase between three and fourfold when close family members suffer from it (Migala, 2022). This has more to do with genetics than the family environment, although this can also influence the likelihood of BPD development.

Coupled with a genetic predisposition toward BPD, living in a stressful, unsupportive environment increases the chances of certain character traits developing into full-blown BPD. Chronic invalidation at home can be problematic, but the thing that often pushes people over the edge is a traumatic event like neglect or abuse. Studies conducted in 2018 revealed that ill-treatment during childhood, including sexual abuse, is a significant risk factor for BPD (Migala, 2022).

Environmental Risk Factors

Experiencing severe trauma in childhood can spark BPD in young adults. People with a genetic predisposition toward BPD may or may not develop the disorder. However, when a traumatic childhood is coupled with genetic factors, the chances of fully-fledged BPD emerging are much greater. Children are transitioning mentally and physically, and this can make them particularly vulnerable to negative experiences, resulting in the development of mental health problems later in life. Risk factors in childhood in vulnerable individuals include:

- emotional, physical, and sexual abuse
- witnessing abuse and domestic violence
- parental neglect
- separation from parents because of desertion or death
  (Kristi, 2020)

These issues significantly raise the risk profiles of those already vulnerable to developing BPD. Between 40% and 86% of people diagnosed with BPD have a history of childhood sexual abuse; 75% were emotionally abused; 75% were physically abused; and 17%–25% experienced severe emotional neglect. When parents and caregivers do not provide a loving, supportive, and safe environment for children, the consequences can be devastating (Kristi, 2020).

Childhood trauma can disrupt the typical development of thoughts and emotions, as well as the ability to identify emotions. Children who experience trauma may have negative perceptions of themselves, others, and relationships. Abused children might develop BPD through insecure attachment. Anxiety plays a role in linking childhood neglect or abuse with BPD. Maternal anxiety and depression during pregnancy can also trigger BPD in offspring. Dysfunctional families, where children become mediators in marital conflicts, or are made to feel guilty for the shortcomings of the adults in their lives and are psychologically controlled, often resulting in BPD symptoms developing in adolescence.

Traumatic early life experiences trigger BPD symptoms like emotional instability, the inability to regulate emotions, and self-harming. This impairs the ability of such children to recognize different emotions and rationalize them. Adverse childhood situations such as parental mental illness, extreme poverty, and emotional and physical trauma were found to be the main contributors to the development of BPD in teens. When such factors combine with a genetic propensity for BPD, there is a high likelihood that this disorder will develop.

Several studies have shown that childhood sexual abuse, together with the associated feelings of depression and a tendency toward substance abuse, is likely to increase the chances of developing severe BPD. Physically abused children manifest a wide range of BPD symptoms. This type of trauma makes it difficult for people to manage their emotions, disturbs their relationships with others, negatively impacts their sense of self, and raises their tendency to self-harm. These individuals are at high risk of developing BPD.

Being bullied and victimized during primary school may raise the likelihood of developing BPD because of the feelings of loneliness, distrust, and fear that this experience engenders. Bullying was found to increase the likelihood of early onset BPD by as much as seven times (Bozzatello et al., 2021).

Some researchers have theorized that impulsivity and reduced emotional control may cause those with BPD to be vulnerable to re-exposure to traumatic events. This further reduces their sense of self and ability to regulate their emotions. They are more likely to see new experiences as threatening and traumatic.

Myth-Busting Borderline Personality Disorder

Because emotional intensity, instability, and unpredictability are the hallmarks of BPD, those who hold the diagnosis are often stigmatized and labeled as abusive, manipulative, dramatic, and self-absorbed. There are several myths surrounding this disorder, and it's necessary to familiarize yourself with them to counter the prevailing misconceptions. This can encourage sufferers to seek support and enable the average person to understand the truth about BPD. Let's unpack some of the more common BPD myths.

Myth #1: Borderline Personality Disorder Justifies Character Flaws

BPD has formally been identified as a mental health disorder accompanied by specific symptoms that are used to make a diagnosis. Internal distress and interpersonal conflict are often experienced by sufferers. While it's rare to diagnose BPD before age 18, symptoms may develop well before then (Terrighena, 2022).

Myth #2: Borderline Personality Disorder is the Same as Schizophrenia or Bipolar Disorder

While some symptoms of BPD might mimic bipolar disorder or schizophrenia, the condition is separate from these diagnoses.

Myth #3: Borderline Personality Disorder is a Female Problem

Three times as many women are diagnosed with BPD than men, but there may be a gender bias inherent in the assessment process (Terrighena, 2022). In fact, BPD is likely to be underdiagnosed in men. BPD symptoms in men are frequently diagnosed as another psychological issue, such as anger management difficulties, addiction, or bipolar disorder. Men and women handle their underlying emotions differently.

Myth #4: Borderline Personality Disorder is Diagnosed in Adults Only

As mentioned previously, BPD is not usually diagnosed in children or young teens, although it may already be developing. Studies have found that over 60% of sufferers experience classic symptoms before the age of 17 (Pattemore, 2021).

Myth #5: People Living with Borderline Personality Disorder are Crazy and Unpredictable

The unpredictable, overreactive behaviors exhibited by people with BPD are their way of coping with tremendous distress. Extreme behaviors result from feelings of anger, fear, stress, cognitive distortions, or an uncertain self-image. These may find an outlet in extreme, impulsive behaviors that seem to come out of nowhere. BPD triggers are often rooted in past negative experiences. Sufferers resort to tactics that worked for them in the past

Myth #6: Borderline Personality Disorder Makes People Dangerous, Abusive, and Manipulative

People with BPD may engage in unhealthy behaviors when they are feeling overwhelmed and have been triggered emotionally. These are usually responses to the powerful emotions they may experience when faced with reminders of times when they felt unsafe, threatened, or when their emotions were unvalidated and they were punished. Their powerful reactions later in life are often trauma responses. People with BPD can learn to regulate their emotions, and the condition should not be an excuse to indulge in toxic behavior patterns. Only 3.5% of violent crimes are tied to mental health, while people who struggle with mental illness are ten times more likely to be the victims of violence than people without a diagnosis (Terrighena, 2022).

Myth #7: People With Borderline Personality Disorder Cannot Form Good Relationships

Once trust and love have evolved in a relationship, people with BPD are highly loyal and trustworthy. They often choose to change and have healthier relationships. Although their fear of abandonment runs deep, these people do not intentionally want to disappoint, hurt, or betray others and only wish to live in a stable, secure, and safe space. They often exhibit high empathy and sensitivity to the needs of others and are active listeners, sensing others' feelings. They are frequently creative, passionate individuals who find an emotional outlet in the creative arts. When someone with BPD is happy, they positively radiate joy. People with BPD frequently build extensive support networks. (Holland,K., Legg, T.J. 2023)

Myth #8: People With Borderline Personality Disorder Are Dramatic Attention-Seekers

While some people with BPD exhibit extreme behaviors like impulsivity, risk-taking, self-harm, and the idealization of suicide, these are not attention-seeking behaviors but attempts to relieve extreme pain. Their emotions are in turmoil, and they are desperate to be understood. When such behaviors elicit angry responses or withdrawal, this makes them more distressed and desperate for understanding. This can lead to conflicts. Their emotions often rule them, and the more rational parts of their brain do not rein them in. Impulsive, risk-taking behaviors often generate guilt and shame.

Myth #9: Borderline Personality Disorder is Untreatable

This is a complete fallacy, as BPD can be treated successfully with different therapies. Schema therapy involves developing schemas or beliefs concerning the individual's worldview, what to expect from others, and what role the self plays in their condition. They learn how to get their basic needs met while improving emotional regulation, self-understanding, and awareness. Cognitive-behavioral therapy (CBT) and Dialectical Behavior Therapy (DBT) are very helpful and effective.

Internalizing Your Knowledge

You will find interactive elements at the end of each chapter containing questions to assist you in reflecting on the relationship you have with someone with BPD. This will enable you to consider how you can use your newfound knowledge to better relate to them.

Consider the following questions:

1. What symptoms of BPD do your loved one, friend, or peer exhibit?
2. How has this impacted your relationship with this individual?

Key Takeaways

BPD is characterized by extreme behaviors, intense mood swings, and often frightening attempts to self-harm. Beneath these outward signs, people with BPD may experience intense emotional pain. BPD is usually diagnosed in early adulthood. While women are diagnosed at higher rates, men can also suffer from BPD. Men are often misdiagnosed because of a known gender bias with current diagnostic tools. The parts of the brain that control emotions are often overdeveloped in people with BPD, whereas those that control rational thought and regulate emotion are underdeveloped. This causes incredibly powerful emotions, which they often struggle to control.

People with BPD are terrified of being abandoned. Many individuals with BPD have experienced childhood neglect, abuse, and severe bullying. Their emotions weren't validated, and they had no outlet to express these intense feelings. There is frequently a genetic history of BPD in families, with children and siblings much more likely to develop BPD if their parents or another sibling holds the diagnosis. BPD is usually diagnosed in young adults, but triggers and symptoms often begin years before.

There are several myths around BPD because it is such an emotive condition, although many have little basis. BPD can be treated successfully with different therapies. People with BPD can form deep, meaningful relationships characterized by passion, creativity and compassion.

In the next chapter, we'll delve deeper into the BPD relationship cycle and the intense underlying emotions.

Chapter 2

An Emotional Rollercoaster: Highs and Lows of Borderline Personality Disorder Relationships

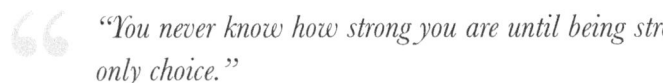 *"You never know how strong you are until being strong is your only choice."*

— Bob Marley

This chapter focuses on how BPD impacts relationships. It's not all bad, however—BPD has positive aspects that can make your relationship more meaningful and fun.

The Borderline Personality Disorder Relationship Cycle

Every relationship has its own specific challenges, so there is no one-size-fits-all approach. Although BPD presents itself differently in everyone, frequent emotional episodes are a reality. No one is superhuman, which means the highs and lows of living with BPD will also affect partners, spouses, friends, and family members. This includes the individuals with BPD's tendency to idealize and then devalue their loved ones, which is referred to as the BPD breakup stages or relationship cycle.

People with BPD often fixate on a particular individual, who becomes their favorite person for a time. This can be a romantic partner, friend, or family member. As such, these chosen people are frequently subjected to this frustrating cycle.

There are seven stages that an individual with BPD may cycle through within their personal relationships.

The Seven Stages of the Borderline Personality Disorder Relationship Cycle

Relationships with individuals with BPD usually go through a cycle of six or seven stages, depending on whether there is a reconciliation after the situation reaches a point of no return (Gilette, 2021).

Stage #1: Attraction

This is the honeymoon stage, where everything is the proverbial sunshine and roses. You are the individual with BPD's favorite person. They adore you and avidly participate in your interests and hobbies. There will often be a powerful attraction created by the people with BPD's habit of mimicking you, which draws you deeper into the relationship. They might make excessive demands on you, but you allow it because you feel this person is "the one," possibly even your soulmate. This phase may persist for up to six months. People drawn into a BPD person's friendship circle often experience something similar, which helps to cement the friendship.

Stage #2: Obsessive Neediness

As the relationship progresses, the individual with BPD may become anxious and fearful, which mystifyingly changes their behavior. They may be unusually irritable about minor annoyances, like delays in responding to texts or calls. If your partner's BPD makes them paranoid, they will believe that these incidents reflect you are not really into them and don't love them. This is brought on by the low self-esteem and terror of abandonment at the heart of BPD.

Stage #3: Withdrawing and Withholding Behaviors

Your BPD partner or friend pushes you away in small ways to see how you respond. This is to force you to satisfy any of their emotional needs that are not being met to their satisfaction. They might instigate "arguments," forcing you to fight for the relationship and, by extension, for them. This is their attempt to feel more secure in themselves and regulate their emotions.

Stage #4: Escalating Devaluation

If your partner or friend with BPD doesn't receive the attention they crave, they panic because what they perceive as a lack of validation triggers their lurking terror of abandonment. They frequently pick fights, the intensity of which escalates. In this phase, people with BPD may devalue their favorite people entirely, painting themselves as victims and even gaslighting their partners or friends. These incidents often come out of nowhere. This combination of behaviors is the main reason many BPD relationships and friendships fail.

Stage #5: The Breakup

The individual with BPD might accuse those they are involved with of being dysfunctional or having a disorder. Once there are no further options for them to pursue, they will abruptly announce that they are breaking up with you—or simply leave without warning. Sometimes, it is because they find another favorite person to hang onto.

As the partner or friend of someone with BPD—even if they are undiagnosed or hide their diagnosis from you—this is often the point where the relationship ends. You might be confused and unable to understand why the relationship is deteriorating and why they have become unrecognizable.

Stage #6: Return and Resolve

If a romantic relationship is relatively new and your BPD partner is still single, they might feel depressed and worthless after the breakup and may contact you to rekindle the relationship. Either way, you decide to take them back, and you might even take the blame for the relationship breakdown. You promise to meet their emotional needs. There might be another shorter honeymoon phase when their dysfunctional behavior ceases for a while. However, the BPD cycle inevitably restarts.

Stage #7: Reconcile and Repeat

It's important to remember that each case is unique. Sometimes, reconciliation will be short-lived, and the situation might become even more explosive than it was before. Your BPD partner might become more manipulative, may gaslight you more intensely, and may have frequent emotional outbursts. They will be triggered more regularly. For the relationship to work, both parties will need to learn how to manage the BPD relationship cycle.

Why Do Borderline Personality Disorder Relationships Cycle?

The BPD relationship cycle is often how the disorder manifests, especially in close relationships. Although it's tremendously difficult to be on the receiving end, the individual with BPD is not deliberately trying to wreck the relationship, nor are they looking for attention. Beneath the drama, they are in considerable emotional distress and pain and are struggling to constrain their emotions. Their self-esteem also wavers. These issues create intense moodiness, characterized by rapid transitions from emotional highs to deep lows. Sometimes, self-sabotage is a way of eliciting the care and attention they crave, particularly if they have accused you of being distant. Behind these behaviors, individuals with BPD are seeking reassurance. While self-sabotage might temporarily resolve their intense emotional turmoil, it can also lead to the cycle repeating continuously.

What to Expect: How Borderline Personality Disorder Affects Relationships

If you are in a relationship with someone with BPD, you know that their mental health issues can make even normal relationship demands significantly more turbulent. Emotional difficulties are more extreme, last longer, and are more challenging to manage than in non-BPD relationships. People with BPD may have trust issues, fear of abandonment, and swing between idealizing and devaluing those close to them. They are hyperaware of anything that might signal rejection and may feel rejected when others do not properly validate their feelings. This perceived rejection often sparks fury that may be out of proportion to the incident that triggered it. The other person might also become angry, escalating the situation.

As discussed previously, the emotional and behavioral manifestations of BPD will affect anyone close to someone with the diagnosis, as well as themselves. They frequently have a record of unhealthy behaviors, instability, and personal relationships characterized by significant conflict. You might be excited about being their favorite person, but when their abandonment issues kick in, there's a good chance they'll leave.

The entire relationship is inherently unstable. You might become uncertain and fearful of setting off bizarre behaviors in your partner or friend. You might wonder if you are cut out for this relationship or friendship. Even when things are relatively good, you might wait apprehensively for the next drama to unfold. This can lead to feelings of guilt, embarrassment, or blaming yourself for their erratic behaviors and moodiness. This is typical of relationships involving someone with BPD.

These relationships can cause trouble, especially when symptoms are severe. The quality of the relationship is often determined by the attitudes and actions of the partner who does not have BPD. Specifically, with romantic relationships, you, as the partner without BPD, will need to decide how much emotional support you will give and how much responsibility you wish to take on to ensure that the relationship perseveres and is successful. Couples therapy can help establish how both partners can support one another, enabling them to express their needs and emotions safely.

People with BPD need to be made aware that they cannot demand more emotional help from others than that person can reasonably give. Many individuals who do not hold a diagnosis also cannot find a middle ground where they can assist those with BPD in their lives without the entire interaction becoming toxic.

All relationships are a two-way street, and the loved one with BPD needs to regulate their emotions themselves with the help of professionals. Partners, spouses, family members, and friends are not therapists and cannot be expected to fulfill a therapeutic role in their relationships with individuals with BPD.

However, if an individual with BPD refuses to admit that there is a problem and does not seek help, then you might want to reconsider your options if you are not obliged to live with them. When a loved one with BPD receives treatment and is surrounded by supportive people, they may sustain good relationships, especially if their symptoms decrease and their emotions stabilize. If they are in therapy, the therapist may want to see their partners, spouses, and family members, too, as this can provide a safe space for you to discuss your feelings and develop the skills to improve the relationship.

Every BPD relationship is unique. The individual may refuse to seek treatment or become destructive and violent. You might not wish to sustain such a relationship or friendship. Especially in the latter case, you may need to cut ties with them for your own well being.

Effects of Borderline Personality Disorder on Families

If a family member exhibits BPD behaviors, diagnosed or not, the entire family can be affected. This is partly because sufferers may create division among family members when they feel frustrated. Very often, such families are predisposed to this because their family dynamics create a situation where there is tremendous conflict and family members are often alienated from one another.

Individuals with BPD may seem more inclined to compete with other family members than work with them. They perceive family resources as being scarce, so they compete for parental favors, approval, attention, or financial resources such as an inheritance.

Another ruse used by individuals with BPD to disrupt positive family interactions is triangulation. This is when a third party is brought into an argument so the two can gang up on the opponent. This can destroy the family structure.

It is important to encourage cooperation by not taking part in the competitions an individual with BPD creates. Consistently encouraging cooperation between family members will strengthen the family structure and its longevity.

There Are Also Positives!

While there are downsides to having a relationship with someone with BPD, there are positives, as well.

- People with BPD are extremely intelligent. They process information and find answers to problems quickly.
- People with BPD know about suffering—their lives have often been filled with loneliness, hurt, and distress. This makes them incredibly compassionate. However, their natural empathy needs to be regulated as they may become burnt out because they identify so strongly with others in difficult situations.
- Individuals with BPD are often emotionally intuitive. They are experts at decoding facial expressions and nonverbal cues, and they are masters at determining the emotional and mental states of others.

- Those individuals with **BPD** who are very motivated to resolve their problems and develop good relationships with others may decide to tackle conflicts head-on. This can be difficult if you prefer to avoid conflict.
- Because they often had dysfunctional childhoods, people with **BPD** might make wonderful parents, as they will do anything to ensure that their children have a better life. If they are prepared to recognize and work on their **BPD**, they can become very responsive, affectionate, and supportive parents.
- People with **BPD** are often seen as fragile, needing protection from life's difficulties. However, they are surprisingly resilient. Despite responding with inappropriate levels of emotion to everyday events, they can be composed and robust during a crisis and will often support their families during difficult times. They are survivors who are frequently a source of strength for others.
- People with **BPD** have tremendous energy and are naturally spontaneous, which can make them very attractive. Their propensity for impulsiveness and risk-taking needs to be channeled positively. For partners and friends, this can create memorable and unique experiences.
- Beneath their symptoms, people with **BPD** have a deep longing for the intimate relationships they have so much trouble maintaining. They are affectionate and passionate and will work hard to deepen their relationships with others. They will compliment you, shower you with affection, and give you plenty of attention. If you can maintain your relationship with a loved one with **BPD**, you are likely to find them becoming more expressive. This might make it easier for

you to open up about your own emotions during difficult times (Lo, 2022).

Cultivating Positive Borderline Personality Disorder Relationships

While a significant number of relationships do not work out for people with BPD, there are some that do.

One of the key requirements for successful relationships is that individuals with BPD need to be committed to therapy and other interventions. Non-BPD partners and family members can become part of the process, for example, by attending therapy sessions when required, and setting reasonable boundaries.

Romantic relationships, where one partner holds a diagnosis of BPD, can also work out well when there is good communication and understanding, and they can talk their way through situations. This rarely happens instantly. Some BPD partners struggle for years before seeing a breakthrough. It can be messy and painful, but eventually, a modicum of equilibrium can be reached with plenty of therapy, love, patience, and the commitment to work on the relationship. Consistent, high-quality therapy and embracing solutions such as DBT are also helpful in reducing emotional intensity so the BPD partner isn't triggered as frequently.

Interactive Element

Consider your current relationship with someone with BPD. Evaluate it using the questions below. Remember, there is no right or wrong answer.

- What are the things you love or enjoy most about this person?
- What traits do you find particularly frustrating and difficult to manage?
- If this person is in therapy, how could you assist them in their journey toward better relationships?

Key Takeaways

While all relationships have their struggles, being close to a loved one with BPD can be challenging. Apart from struggling to control the emotional rollercoaster without being sucked into it themselves, partners, friends, and family members may also need to cope with the BPD relationship cycle, which can feel more like a fatal attraction. The cycle usually includes the following stages:

- powerful attraction
- obsessive neediness
- withdrawing and withholding behaviors
- devaluing those close to them, including gaslighting, lying, and painting themselves as the victim
- breaking up, often suddenly and unexpectedly
- return and resolution
- reconciliation and a repeat of the cycle

Relationships with individuals with BPD can be extremely intense and require tremendous emotional commitment. Everyone needs support, and it's essential that those who do not hold the diagnosis take time to care for their own personal needs.

People with BPD are often highly intelligent, adventurous people with tremendous energy. They are highly empathetic, emotionally intuitive, and good listeners who often make excellent parents. Being in a relationship with them can be very positive.

Maintaining close relationships with people with BPD can work but may require high levels of commitment. Some sources suggest that people living with BPD might be better off with introverts or other people with BPD, who are better able to understand their struggles.

In the next chapter, you'll find out how to communicate effectively with someone close to you who has BPD.

Chapter 3

Effective Communication Strategies

 "There is hope, even if your brain tells you there isn't."

—John Green

Communication is the foundation of all good relationships, and the same applies to those where one party holds the diagnosis of BPD. In this chapter, you'll discover different communication strategies that could enable you to be more empathetic while de-escalating difficult situations.

Validating Feelings

Validation is the art of affirming another, putting yourself in their shoes, and accepting their emotions, feelings, and thoughts as understandable and valid under the circumstances. This does not mean agreeing with them, complimenting them, forgetting about boundaries, or trying to change their minds. Validating someone with BPD means actively listening, hearing, and accepting them.

Validation has several benefits, including:

- encouraging and supporting positive change
- helping people with BPD acknowledge the reality and logic of their own experience
- promoting emotional equilibrium
- improving relationships, encouraging intimacy, and building trust
- helping individuals trust their feelings
- encouraging them to listen to you because they feel you understand their perspective
- helping individuals with BPD feel more connected
- your own validation (Garlan, 2016)

Dangers of Invalidating Borderline Personality Disorder Individuals

When you invalidate individuals with BPD, you ignore, reject, or judge their emotional experiences. If you delay validation because you are waiting until you understand them better, you are effectively telling them that their emotional responses need to be the same as yours. This means you value control more than emotional displays, so people with BPD may find it even harder to regulate their feelings. Such attitudes can also be very hurtful.

Invalidating actions may include:

- brushing off or trivializing someone else's experiences
- blaming or name-calling
- telling someone to "let it go" or "get over it"
- trying to solve someone's problems before having all the information

- having inappropriate body language or facial expressions (Garlan, 2016)

Because intense emotion is so much a part of the way a loved one with BPD sees the world, your rejection of their emotions, thoughts, or experiences is often taken personally. It's important to be mindful so you don't invalidate your loved one. They may feel that you are judging them negatively if you reach a particular conclusion about a situation. If you convey by your actions or responses that their emotional expression is flawed, they might struggle to trust themselves, which inhibits their ability to make decisions, solve problems, or act. This creates a form of "learned helplessness."

Why Is Validation Difficult?

Validation can be difficult when you see the situation solely from your own perspective. You might find the emotional displays of an individual with BPD unsettling or frightening. Remember, what is happening is not about you. You don't need to understand, agree with, be comfortable with, or react to their behavior.

Communicating with a very emotional individual with BPD can be overwhelming. You may experience anger, fear, or resentment. You may worry that validation will escalate the situation rather than ease it. Your instinct may be to fix what is wrong. You may wish that the reality was different. If you haven't done your research, you may not know much about BPD.

Tips for Effective Validation

- Be sensitive and take it slowly. If they feel you got it wrong, then acknowledge this.

- Only emotions need validation.
- Remain calm and reflect back to them what they just said. Keep a neutral tone, and don't have any expectations. Allow your tone to show that you may have it wrong.
- Listen to what is not being said. Note their facial expressions and body language. Consider what you know about them.
- Look at the person's feelings in the light of their past and reflect this back to them to show that you appreciate where they are coming from.
- Show that their experience is valid, given common experiences for people in that situation.
- Demonstrate that you are on the same level and don't act superior. Don't treat them as fragile or incompetent. Empathize—give them a hug, apologize if you made a mistake, and hand them tissues or cry with them when they are upset.

Validation Tips

Do	Don't
Listen with your full attention— make eye contact and lean in. Look and act interested.	Don't respond emotionally, as this will escalate the situation.
Listen to the feelings behind the words.	Don't appeal to their logic. Those with BPD won't respond to this.
Listen to their needs.	Don't give them ultimatums. This makes it appear that you aren't listening to them and don't understand their feelings.
	Don't dominate the situation—this is very invalidating for those with BPD. It makes them stressed and worsens the situation. Control your responses.
	Don't fix things. It's important that an individual with BPD finds their own solutions.

Validating individuals with BPD reduces their emotional intensity. Getting it wrong means that the situation might escalate, or they could shut down completely. It takes time to learn to validate properly, so keep working on it. Avoid judging or blaming yourself. Release past hurts and disappointments. Being afraid, exhausted, and overwhelmed can make validation more difficult.

Reducing Borderline Rage

Borderline rage refers to the unbridled fury that manifests in individuals with borderline personality disorder. It may be sparked by a seemingly trivial event or occur randomly. This is what therapists refer to as "challenging behavior." In people with BPD, this is uncontrollable anger that may put their partners, families, and themselves at risk of psychological or physical harm. They may become destructive, breaking objects around them. Their rage often has severe repercussions for themselves and their partners, families, and social circle.

If you are on the receiving end of these tirades, you might wonder how long it's going to continue and could become frightened if their anger becomes violent, whether directed at you, other people, or material objects. The episodes may last anywhere from a few hours to a few days, depending on the individual and the severity of their symptoms.

Causes of Borderline Personality Disorder Rage

People with BPD struggle with situations that annoy them or that they find stressful, which might spark their anger. Some causes include:

- As mentioned previously, people with BPD have intense, often negative, emotional responses to events. They interpret the world differently from neurotypical individuals and may feel threatened by seemingly trivial things. They find it difficult to regulate their emotions, impulsivity, and hostility.
- Their fear of abandonment is another complication. While many welcome time alone, for people with BPD, this is an excruciating prospect. If they believe, often erroneously, that they are about to be abandoned, they will go into a blind panic, which manifests as anger.

- The tendency of individuals with BPD to see everything in black-and-white terms is referred to as "BPD splitting." Positive experiences stimulate and excite them, while perceived negative ones can quickly cause frustration, disappointment, or even disgust. This may generate uncontrollable anger, and the individual with BPD "splits."
- Many people suffering from mental disorders or illnesses experience anger and frustration. Specifically, those with BPD often brood on their anger, which stokes the fire. This can make them more aggressive, creating a cycle of rage. People with BPD may get angrier more often, more intensely, and for longer periods than a neurotypical person (Antonatos, 2022).

Tips for Managing Borderline Personality Disorder Anger

For Individuals with BPD

- Anger may lurk in the background, coming out of nowhere to hijack you when you least expect it. You need to recognize that you are becoming angry so you can take steps to control it. For example, anger might generate physical manifestations, like feeling hot and sweaty, having tense muscles, or a racing heartbeat.
- You need to identify what triggers your anger. Fury is often caused by misinterpreting situations or others' actions. Pinpointing the reasons for your anger will help you mitigate it before it controls you. Those close to you can assist by helping to identify your triggers in an objective, non-threatening, and conciliatory way.

- Another helpful way to deal with BPD anger is to interrupt the process by distracting yourself so you stop focusing on your anger. This can include exercises like going for a walk or run, playing soothing, calming music, or doing something enjoyable, like a favorite hobby, cooking, or something creative.
- You can also do deep, mindful breathing and try to think about things you find calming and relaxing. Try to do this as soon as the anger emerges to avoid having an extended anger episode. Doing progressive muscle relaxation techniques can also help.
- Avoid bottling up your emotions, as this may drive your feelings underground, where they become more intense, gradually building, increasing tension, and often breeding resentment. It is important to acknowledge and address your feelings and speak up early. Becoming assertive might be difficult, but it is a skill that can be practiced and learned.
- Lower your stress levels, as stress and anger are often linked. Alert the people you are close to when you are becoming stressed and ask them to help you mitigate your stress.

Tips for Partners, Friends, and Family

Those close to individuals with BPD need to adopt effective verbal communication skills to de-escalate situations involving BPD rage. Strategies include:

- Remain calm and objective so you can assess the situation and respond appropriately.
- Listen actively, offering the person your attention,

acknowledging their emotions, and focusing on establishing where the problem lies.

- Always use positive language and avoid negativity.
- Be open when communicating with the person so you gain their trust, and they can calm down (*Responding to Challenging Behavior*, 2018).

Using "I" Statements

When you are in a conflict situation, it's sometimes difficult to express your feelings without making things worse. Using "I" messages—assertiveness statements—means you can voice your feelings and concerns in such a way that the other person finds them acceptable. Using "I" statements reflects your own experiences and emotions without focusing on what the other person has done or not done. You can, therefore, express yourself without attacking, blaming, or criticizing others. This neutralizes hostility, defensiveness, and conflict. "I" messages create a window for constructive, open discussions about the reasons your partner was so upset.

While they won't solve all your problems, using "I" messages improves assertiveness and resolves conflict more effectively, creating opportunities for constructive feedback. They enable you to explain how things appear from your point of view. "I" messages are primarily intended to:

- be clear rather than polite
- state how the situation looks from your perspective
- allow you to explain how you would like things to be
- open up healthy conversations so problems can be resolved (Montemurro, 2011)

Remember that "I" messages won't elicit the responses you would like, they simply enable you to voice your feelings in an acceptable way. Expecting others to comply with your wishes without delay is unrealistic. You can't force them to remedy the problem by simply using "I" messages.

The Four Parts of an "I" Message

An "I" message usually:

- begins by identifying your emotions and feelings, e.g., "I feel angry"
- mentions what you are upset about—what someone said or did
- explains why you feel this way, e.g., "I have asked you to do this several times," or "That embarrassed me"
- explains what you'd prefer to happen, e.g., "Can we please keep our problems to ourselves?" (Montemurro, 2011)

Examples of "You" Messages Versus "I" Messages

"You" Messages	"I" Messages
You never put anything away. The house looks like a dump.	I feel annoyed when I come home, and everything is all over the place.
You're always embarrassing me — you did it at dinner last night, too.	I felt really embarrassed when we were at Tony's the other night, and we were talking about this because...
You said you'd text me, but you didn't.	I get worried when I don't hear from you. I just want to be sure that you are safe.
You never listen to anyone, and you're not listening to me now.	I feel my concerns are not being heard.
You never tell me how you are feeling.	I would love to know how you feel about this.
I hate when you yell and swear at the kids.	When you shout at the kids, I get annoyed because I feel they should be treated with respect. Please don't yell or swear at them.
You are always late. It's rude, and you mess up everybody else's schedules.	When you start work half an hour later than you're supposed to, I feel frustrated because we can't start our meetings on time. I would prefer that you arrive at work at 8:30, as that's what we agreed upon.

Confronting Conflict

We have all heard the saying that sticks and stones will break your bones, but words will never harm you. The truth is that words can, and do, wound. Individuals with BPD often argue with others for the sake of arguing. It is frustrating to be on the receiving end.

Poor Conflict Strategies: An Example

Rose, who is diagnosed with BPD, complains to her boyfriend, Alec, about her friend Diana. She accuses Diana of being deceitful and hypercritical. When Alec asks for clarification, Rose becomes angry. She gets even angrier and switches to defending her friend when Alec tells her she's being unrealistic.

Alec sometimes joins in when Rose gets angry, venting his own frustrations. This only adds fuel to the proverbial fire. At other times, Alec himself engages in manipulative behavior, drinking excessively or refusing to go to work, blaming his behavior on Rose's inability to control her emotions. He sometimes tries to humor her out of her annoyance, saying that their conversation was ridiculous. Rose, honing in on her emotions, cannot appreciate his attempts at levity. Instead, she feels trivialized and dismissed.

A better approach for Alec would be to encourage Rose to express her feelings rather than being quick to voice his own opinions and suggestions. If he can do this in such a way as to avoid escalating the conflict, possibly by using "I" statements, Alec could make Rose aware of the hurtfulness of her own words or behavior. This will enable Rose to step back and take responsibility.

Arguing Constructively

Individuals with BPD are very sensitive and will notice when you're just going through the motions of listening. As children, they were often ignored or dismissed. If you make a genuine effort, this will make them calmer. Remember to validate their feelings. You don't need to have all the answers.

Some people with BPD may have been severely traumatized as children. Consider that you're not arguing with an adult but dealing with a child in severe emotional pain. By noting their body language and tone of voice, you observe them regressing back to a traumatized child. This will help you understand their actions. Lashing out is the reaction of a child who doesn't know how to handle a situation.

It might be hard to take a step back, especially if you're feeling resentful or being shouted at, but do your best to see the wounded child hiding behind the person's behavior and be compassionate. Look beyond what they are saying in order to see their unmet needs. These could be something current or a hang-over from the past.

Remember that you aren't responsible for the entire relationship. Balance healthy boundaries with empathy, being loving but firm. You might not get into the reasons for setting boundaries during a fierce argument. Avoid walking away if you can—this will inflame the fears of abandonment—but hold your ground. Say things like, "I don't want to, but if you continue to... I will need to..." or "I can understand how you feel, and I will do... for you, but I won't tolerate..."

Once their inner child is subdued and they are calmer, discuss their triggers and what you can do or refrain from doing so that things don't escalate. Reach a middle ground where everyone's needs are met.

You can't save them and should not blame yourself for being unable to change their past or their genes. This can create an unhealthy dynamic, and your relationship may deteriorate. Be warm and compassionate, but ensure that they remain responsible for their own personal growth. Being with someone who has

BPD is difficult, but they have many positive attributes that can make the relationship worthwhile.

If their symptoms are severe, you can't work things out, or the situation becomes dangerous, you are not obliged to stay. However, if you decide to stay and it is safe for you to do so, then your commitment could help place them on the road to recovery.

Trying to Fix Things

Everyone needs emotional support and practical help, and what better way to receive this than in a healthy relationship? However, it's necessary to establish which option is appropriate for a situation. To achieve the right balance between listening and helping, it's necessary to do the following:

- Understand both yourself and the individual with BPD, evaluate the results of your actions, and learn from your mistakes.
- Recognize that everyone has legitimate needs.
- Manage your feelings and express them calmly, being careful to avoid criticism, hostility, and impulsiveness (Davila, 2016).

Recognize that you are an individual and look for support in different ways. Focus on understanding both perspectives and allow the individual with BPD to express their feelings, too. This will soothe their pain, and they might even take the actions you have suggested.

Doing the same things repeatedly won't generate a different result. Insisting on a particular solution can make those with BPD feel unheard and misunderstood. They might blame you for the impasse. If something doesn't work, stop doing it. If they prefer emotional support, don't focus only on physical support, but give them what they need. If they are problem solvers, allow them to provide this type of support, as it will validate them and make them feel they are important to you.

Talk about the support you need, as well as what you could provide. Focus on solving problems together rather than pitting yourselves against each other. This is not what individuals with BPD need. If you truly care about the other person, then offer the right type of support. Focus on the compassion and empathy you have for the loved one with BPD rather than the frustration and anger you may sometimes feel. Stay with them through their pain, listen, and provide the right type of support rather than arguing.

Interactive Element: Dealing With Conflict

Because conflict is common in relationships with individuals with BPD, it's helpful to reflect on solutions that might assist you. Read through this chapter again and have a notepad and pen handy. Jot down three things from this chapter that you could put into practice in your relationship. Try to use these pointers whenever the need arises. Mentally notice the difference it makes when you use these strategies.

Not all the strategies will work immediately—they aren't magic—and some won't work at all. Try different approaches over a period of time to establish which are most effective.

Key Takeaways

Being in a relationship with someone with BPD can be explosive, as they are hyperaware and can be triggered by even small occurrences. Anger is often their response, sometimes born of frustration, but very often the result of their traumatized inner child coming to the forefront. Effective communication is key to calming the borderline's erratic, emotional behavior.

Validating their emotions is very important. This doesn't mean agreeing with them or condoning their destructive behavior but acknowledging their right to feel their emotions. There are several ways in which you can validate their emotions. This helps to calm fraught situations and promotes feelings of connection rather than fear of abandonment.

When you have someone with BPD in your life, conflict resolution skills are essential. They have very little control over their anger. It's important to ensure that it doesn't boil over into uncontrolled rage that could last for days, culminating in frightening, wild behaviors.

Avoid getting embroiled in the argument. Listen actively to establish what's really going on. To de-escalate the situation, suggest that they take time out by deep breathing, doing progressive relaxation techniques, going for a walk or another form of exercise, and doing things they enjoy. This will prevent them from dwelling on their angry thoughts and spiraling out of control. Remain compassionate, remembering that there's a hurt, traumatized child hiding behind the façade but remember to affirm your boundaries.

It's helpful to use "I" statements when facing an argument. This enables you to express your feelings calmly without resorting to criticism, blame, or hostility. It's important to discuss things when they have calmed down to establish what type of support they need. Tell them what support you need as well. People with BPD are often natural empaths and would welcome the chance to help.

Setting boundaries is essential, as there need to be certain behaviors for which you have a zero-tolerance approach to ensure the health of the relationship and your own mental well-being. In the next chapter, you'll discover how to approach this thorny issue effectively and safely.

Chapter 4

Setting Boundaries Without Building Walls

"I keep moving ahead, as always, knowing deep down inside that I am a good person, and that I am worthy of a good life."

— Jonathan Harnisch

This chapter explains how you can set healthy boundaries with individuals with BPD. This is essential, as you will often be required to put up with extreme and often disrespectful behavior to "prove" you love and care for them. Here, you will find some tips to enable you to set these boundaries in such a way as to affirm their feelings without feeling guilty yourself.

The Importance of Setting Healthy Boundaries

Boundaries, as the name implies, are limits you set with other people to assert your needs and wants without being aggressive. Boundaries usually apply to behaviors that make you feel uncomfortable or disrespected. Having boundaries prevents others from taking advantage of you, which can make you resentful. It's important to speak up when others behave in unacceptable ways so they know where your boundaries lie.

Setting boundaries doesn't mean that you never need to compromise or that you can have your own way all the time. It simply means that you ensure others respect you. If you don't set boundaries, you may be implicitly agreeing to things that make you uncomfortable or stressed. You might burn out as you struggle to meet everyone's demands on your time and resources. Burnout can also cause stress and anxiety, so it's important to set limits.

When you set boundaries with others, this means that you have better relationships with them because you don't get resentful and can be clear about your needs and resources.

The Difficulty of Setting Boundaries with Individuals with Borderline Personality Disorder

A lack of boundaries often characterizes relationships where one person holds a BPD diagnosis. Neurotypical partners, families, and friends may give in to their demands, sometimes becoming so enmeshed that lines are blurred. Without proper boundaries, people with BPD risk sacrificing others' strength and individuality.

Constantly interacting with someone with BPD can be very tiring and demanding. Setting firm boundaries will help to maintain your mental well-being, making it less likely you become resentful, angry, overwhelmed, and burned out.

Unfortunately, people with BPD may find boundaries offensive, which is one reason their relationships risk becoming unstable and unsatisfactory. If you want to be emotionally intimate with someone, you need to set boundaries with them and respect their boundaries as well. This ensures that everyone feels safe and comfortable. When you are in a relationship with someone who has BPD, they will continually test your boundaries.

When you attempt to set boundaries with them, they will resist because they feel rejected. They have the erroneous belief that if you love them, you will "prove" it by tolerating their negative, antisocial behavior. Ignoring specifically defined boundaries is one of the main ways people with BPD get others to "prove" their love for them. If you relax a boundary, they will continue to violate it, presuming that you will relax other boundaries you might have put in place as well. This might leave you feeling that nothing is off limits for them and that it's useless to set boundaries.

Tips for Setting Boundaries with Individuals with Borderline Personality Disorder

When setting boundaries with an individual with BPD, you need to ensure that they are:

- Explicitly clear. For example, if you do not want them to call you after a certain time of night, state your exact cut-off time for calls.
- Consistency is extremely important.
- Presented calmly, or they will feel justified in flouting them and might play the victim (*Why is Setting Boundaries*, 2017).

Defining Boundaries

What Boundaries Are	What Boundaries Are Not
Determined by us.	Set for us by others.
Clear and firm	Manipulative or controlling
Protective	Hurtful or harmful
Flexible	Immovable and rigid
Appropriate and receptive	Dominating or invasive

Types of Boundaries

There are several types of boundaries. Here are some examples:

- *Nonnegotiable boundaries* concern your safety. This includes protection from domestic violence and substance abuse, as well as life-threatening health issues and partner infidelity. Don't make too many of your boundaries nonnegotiable, and be prepared to enforce them.
- *Physical boundaries* protect your body and personal space, both of which belong to you. These include things such as whether you like to be touched, how close you like people to be to you, your privacy, and your physical needs.
- *Sexual boundaries* refer to your consent, your right to determine what sexual encounters you prefer, how often you want to have sex, where, and with whom.
- *Emotional boundaries* can be defined as the right to have your own thoughts and emotions, as well as taking

responsibility for them. This means not over-sharing, being appropriate, and respecting the feelings of others.

- *Time boundaries* refer to your choice of how you spend your time. These protect you from overwork or giving too much of your time to a particular person, cause, or activity.
- *Spiritual or religious boundaries* respect your right to believe in whatever deity you prefer, worship as you wish, and practice your beliefs—or be agnostic or atheist.
- *Financial or material boundaries* concern your rights over your money and possessions. They mean you can spend your money as you wish, give to charities, or loan money to others. It also means that you may be paid for the work you do (Martin, 2020).

Setting and Maintaining Clear Boundaries

People with BPD often engage in impulsive, self-destructive behaviors that can be harmful to them and others. It's essential that you never validate these inappropriate reactions or behaviors, for example, by giving in to them when they threaten suicide or self-harm. Doing so makes it very difficult to establish boundaries.

You don't need to feel guilty or uncomfortable, apologize, or offer any explanations when you say no. You can have reasonable boundaries in place and still help others. You can validate an individual with BPD while remaining firm in setting behavioral limits.

Make sure that you are utterly certain about your decision, especially if you feel the boundary you are about to set will trigger an individual with BPD. Personal boundaries are not negotiable. As mentioned previously, once you waver on a boundary you have set, this will open the door to all your boundaries being violated.

When saying no, ensure that you have a valid reason for your decision and that you are respectful and empathetic. This sends a message that you have considered their request but that you also have limitations. Practice saying "that doesn't work for me" in a calm, straightforward, kind way.

Attempt to reassure the person that you are not rejecting them when you say no or set a boundary. Reassure them you love them and mention your appreciation of their positive traits. If they are still upset, consider an alternative that meets both your needs to show them you care about them.

Remember not to take reactions personally, as failing to stay calm can escalate the situation. Focus on the issue and avoid being judgmental. You can acknowledge their feelings without condoning their poor behavior.

Boundaries and Emotional Detachment: What's the Difference?

Emotional detachment is when someone distances themselves from the emotions of others. This may be because of a short-term difficulty, such as a stressful situation or an underlying psychological problem. It can be useful for setting boundaries, particularly with people who demand too much of your emotional attention.

However, emotional detachment can be detrimental when it happens spontaneously, making you feel muted. This can show an underlying psychological condition that may require professional intervention.

Symptoms of emotional detachment include:

- lack of commitment to people or relationships
- appearing preoccupied when around others
- inability to express emotions properly
- reduced empathy
- avoiding places, people, or situations associated with past trauma
- withholding emotions or feelings from others
- finding difficulty being affectionate or loving with family members
- not making others a priority when they should be
- experiencing feelings of emptiness or lack of emotion
- being harsh or unkind (Lawrenz, 2023)

Emotional detachment can be deliberate, for example, when someone purposely withdraws from an emotional situation or refuses to engage with someone who habitually upsets them. This is usually a protective measure.

It can also be caused by traumatic events, including abuse or neglect during childhood, when emotional detachment becomes a survival mechanism. In its most extreme form, this may present as reactive attachment disorder (RAD), where children become incapable of bonding with their parents or caregivers. This can lead to emotional or behavioral problems.

Guilt-Free Boundary Setting

Many people feel guilty or uncomfortable when setting boundaries with others. This is normal, especially when you aren't in the habit of doing it. Being unable to say no sets you up for disappointment, frustration, resentment, stress, and burnout.

Unless you get accustomed to setting boundaries, nothing will change.

Setting healthy boundaries isn't selfish, although it focuses on your preferences within relationships and what you will and won't tolerate. Healthy boundaries ensure others are not taking more than you can reasonably give to them, irrespective of how it might make them feel. If you are focused on being nice, then the chances are that you will set weak boundaries, helping others out of a sense of obligation rather than kindness. You're also more likely to feel guilty about setting boundaries if you're inclined to be a people pleaser.

Avoid setting boundaries when you are feeling uncertain, anxious, or angry—and set them early in the relationship before your resentment and frustration build. This often sabotages attempts to set boundaries and results in arguments. Set them when you are calm and able to have a rational discussion with a person so you can consider their point of view. When calm you're more likely to be compassionate, reducing the hurt they might feel.

You may need a fresh perspective to understand why you find it so difficult to set boundaries. You might try to be "nice" to keep the peace while your frustration and resentment simmer. Step back mentally, imagining yourself as an observer. Why are you allowing people to treat you as though you don't matter? Face your feelings and stop avoiding your emotions. Then, set your boundaries, even if it doesn't make you popular.

It's helpful to spend time with people who are comfortable setting boundaries with others. This will enable you to see boundary-setting in perspective, perceiving that limitations are beneficial for healthy relationships. People who care about each other don't run off when another person establishes a boundary.

Don't apologize for setting boundaries—this makes the effort appear half-hearted, and those on the receiving end won't take you seriously. Don't tolerate unacceptable behavior for a long period and then set extreme boundaries when your patience runs out. This can be a hurtful surprise for the person on the receiving end. You should, however, apologize if you were wrong and have needlessly upset the other person.

What happens if it's the person with BPD in your life who is making you feel guilty about setting boundaries? Even if they start off by reacting negatively, they should adapt if they really care about you and the relationship. You can also confirm how important your relationship is to you when you set a boundary. It's helpful to remember your reasons for setting the boundary in the first place—to protect yourself and ensure that they respect you and acknowledge what you need from them.

Interactive Element: Taking Action

After reading this chapter, consider the boundaries you would like to set with people in your life, specifically the person with BPD. Consider how you can approach this issue with them. Ask yourself the following questions:

- Which of their behaviors do you find disrespectful, overwhelming, or frustrating?
- What are three areas where you would like to set boundaries with them?
- How could you approach this conversation in a calm, empathetic manner?

Key Takeaways

In many types of relationships, it's important to set boundaries to avoid being disrespected, overwhelmed, burnt out, and taken for granted. This is not selfish; it's essential to protect your mental and emotional well-being. There are many types of boundaries, including physical, sexual, emotional, time, spiritual, and financial.

It's often difficult to set boundaries when you are with someone with BPD, as doing so is likely to be misconstrued as rejection. They may have an intense dislike of boundary-setting, as they expect you to "prove" your love for them by not having boundaries. This means that they can call on you at any time for anything they might need or desire. This can be very exhausting and may infringe on your personal space, your privacy, and fulfilling your own needs.

It's essential to set boundaries to ensure that you do not become responsible for someone else's emotions, thoughts, or actions. For this to be effective, do this only when you are calm. Ensure that you are clear about the boundaries you wish to set and stick with them. Allowing anyone, including people with BPD, to violate your boundaries means they will continue to do so with impunity.

It's important that you validate them and reiterate the importance of your relationship when you do this. Never apologize for setting a boundary, and don't take their response personally. You may, however, feel guilty about setting boundaries, especially if you are not used to doing this, are inclined to be a people pleaser, or find it hard to say no. There are several strategies you can use to overcome this guilt, enabling you to have healthier, happier relationships. Another way of doing this is to deliberately detach yourself emotionally while setting boundaries so that the person's reaction has little effect on you.

In the next chapter, you will discover how to draw the line between compassion and codependency so you can care for the person in your life with BPD while protecting your own emotional and mental well-being.

Reaching Out to Others

"I think we forget sometimes how blessed we are to be able to help others and make a difference!"

— Gautam Rode

No matter the relationship you have with the person in your life with Borderline Personality Disorder, it's been affecting you. That's why you're here now reading this.

The purpose of this book is to give you the tools you need to support the person you care about while taking care of your own needs. But there are other people out there like you, and the goal of Freeman Publishing is to reach as many of them as possible. If we can do that, we can help not only the people who are living alongside BPD; we can help those who are navigating it themselves, too.

And this is where you come in. Help us reach more of those people who are looking for support through the simple act of leaving your feedback online.

By leaving a review of this book on Amazon, you will help other people looking for guidance for dealing with a friend, family member, co-worker or loved one with BPD find the information they're looking for.

People are looking for support, just as you were. You can help them to find the footing they so desperately need.

Thank you for your support. You know how important this is, better than anyone.

Scan the QR code below for a quick review!

Chapter 5

Compassion Versus Codependency
—Finding the Balance

"Even the darkest night will end, and the sun will rise."

— Victor Hugo, *Les Miserables*

In this chapter, you'll discover what a codependent relationship is and how it can impact family and romantic relationships, especially when one person has BPD. You'll also find out about coping strategies, as well as things you can do to strengthen your relationship.

What is Codependency?

Codependency is an unhealthy attachment between two people, where one person is needy, and the other needs to be needed.

A codependent person is the giver, while the other is the taker. This is not the normal give-and-take found in healthy relationships, where taking responsibility for others is usually balanced with taking responsibility for oneself. Codependency creates very unequal relationships that are usually weighed in favor of the taker. The giver is forced to give without respite, often at a significant cost to themselves. Codependency often destroys the possibility of genuine relationships with others.

Some people are more likely to become codependent because of the following reasons:

- The prefrontal cortex, the rational part of the brain, may not sufficiently regulate empathetic responses.
- Changes in the way society views gender roles or familial substance abuse can foster codependence.
- Some people are more inclined by nature to care for others (Gould, 2022).

The Link Between Borderline Personality Disorder and Codependency

It's easy to become codependent when someone close to you has BPD. Codependency means that you are sacrificing a disproportionate amount of your time, along with your own wants and needs, to maintain an often unhealthy relationship. Your sense of self-worth may become rooted in the fact that you are the responsible and stable person in the relationship. Codependency arises in those who rely on others to generate their sense of self-worth.

People with BPD may also be codependent, although this stems from their fear of abandonment and determination to avoid that possibility at all costs. For individuals with BPD, codependency may cause relationship addiction, creating one-sided, abusive, or emotionally destructive relationships. Family members or couples often refuse to discuss or acknowledge the person's disorder. This can be denial, where help is neither sought nor welcomed because they don't want to admit that the problem exists.

When an individual with BPD is codependent, they may be manipulative, controlling, resentful, overly responsible, and self-pitying. They may try to influence the giver's behavior by manipulating or controlling them, using tactics such as stonewalling or threatening self-harm or suicide. Because they are doing so much for others, they might feel resentful, unappreciated, and self-pitying. They might even burn out.

The giver may find it hard to extricate themselves from the relationship once this pattern is established because they believe that the other person relies on them completely. The taker might also find it difficult to leave what is essentially a toxic relationship because they rely significantly on the giver.

Differentiating Between Compassion and Codependency

Not knowing the difference between compassion and codependency means that those trapped in unhealthy, addictive relationships might not recognize it and break free. When you have compassion, you perceive an individual and their choices lovingly, accepting them without judgment while maintaining healthy boundaries. Codependency is different. Fear is the basis of these relationships. Those involved refuse to accept that the other person has the freedom to make their own choices and live their own lives. They are concerned about how this would affect them and their relationship. Codependency attempts to control the choices of others.

Loving someone means allowing them to be free to make their own choices. Trying to control them stifles both your life journey and that of the other person. A relationship based on control and fear rather than freedom and love means that neither person becomes who they are supposed to be.

Signs of Codependency

If you're unsure whether you are codependent, some indicators include:

- trying to change or rescue people with deep-seated emotional problems that are beyond your capacity to remedy
- idolizing the other person, even if they don't deserve it
- doing whatever the other person demands, even if you are not comfortable with it
- only feeling good about yourself when others like you
- feeling that you need to check in with the other person or request their permission to do routine tasks
- doing anything to avoid conflict with the other person, so you always feel as though you are tiptoeing around them
- feeling sorry for the other person, even when you're the one they've hurt
- often apologizing, even when you've done nothing wrong
- spending all your free time on the other person so you have no time for yourself
- feeling as though you've lost yourself in the relationship (Gould, 2022)

How to Stop Being Codependent

If you feel you tick the boxes for being codependent, there are several things you can do to break the cycle.

Discover Your Attachment Style

As we grow up, we form bonds with others, and our early relationships with our parents and caregivers can influence how we bond with others in the future. These are known as attachment styles. There are four different types (Dodgson, 2023).

Secure Attachment

Most people fall into this category. When they were infants and young children, their parents or caregivers met all their needs, which made them feel comfortable and secure. As adults, such people are comfortable giving their partners personal freedom. They accept their shortcomings and provide for their needs. Secure people have good self-esteem and don't manipulate other people or play games. Their conflict-resolution skills are effective and healthy.

Anxious Attachment

This attachment style develops when young children have unpredictable caregivers, where love and support alternate with dismissiveness or even cruelty. These people have difficulty expressing their needs and emotions. They may become borderline codependent, needing constant affirmation and love. They crave predictability and may cling to the people they are closest to, fearing abandonment. They might play games, withdraw, or try to make others jealous.

Avoidant-Dismissive and Fearful-Avoidant

As the names suggest, people with these attachment styles do their best to avoid relationships altogether and might leave new relationships quickly through fear of abandonment. They were often "perfect" children who rarely complained and simply assumed that their needs would not be met. They rarely trust others and prefer to keep to themselves. There are two forms of avoidant attachment styles:

- *Avoidant-dismissive people avoid emotional closeness.* They distance themselves emotionally from their partners and the important people in their lives, which makes them appear self-centered.
- *Fearful-avoidant people crave closeness but also fear it.* This creates messy, confused, and ambivalent relationships. They don't want to get too close or become too distant from others. They struggle with emotional regulation, frequently becoming overwhelmed, and have intense mood swings.

Insecure attachment styles like the last three often make people fear abandonment. Identifying your attachment style can help you understand how you behave in relationships so that you can avoid codependent tendencies and behaviors. For example, if you grew up in a home where there was substance abuse or constant conflict, you could have an anxious attachment style, increasing your chances of becoming codependent.

Improving Your Self-Esteem

Codependency is often triggered by poor self-esteem, which can make it difficult to set boundaries, stand up for yourself, and articulate your needs. Affirm your positive attributes, as this will automatically raise your feelings of self-worth. Recognize your strengths, setting aside time for things that matter to you.

Focusing on Personal Growth

Growing as a person reduces your need for codependency. Self-improvement enables you to perceive your own value and develop your personal strengths. This helps you create a satisfying life that doesn't depend on others for validation. Evaluate your life and set some future goals. Focus on developing supportive, nurturing relationships.

Improving Your Communication Skills

Communication is the glue that holds all close relationships together. Being a good communicator helps you articulate your needs clearly, reducing codependency. Ask open-ended questions to encourage others to open up about their thoughts and feelings rather than guessing. Set aside time to communicate with the important people in your life so you can discuss any concerns.

Cultivating "Me" Time

The best way to move away from being codependent is to take small steps to become more independent. These may include taking time for yourself, reconnecting with old friends, finding activities you enjoy doing alone, and connecting with new people.

Support Versus Enabling

Being close to someone who has BPD means there is a fine line between supporting them and enabling their behaviors. Being supportive means doing something for another person who cannot do it for themselves, like looking after their children while they are in the hospital. Enabling is doing things for another person who can and should do it for themselves.

Enabling someone with BPD means they are protected from the consequences of their actions. They might not acknowledge that they have a problem, receive treatment, or reach their personal potential. There is no motivation for them to address their disorder, and they become increasingly dependent on you.

Individuals with BPD are often in considerable emotional pain. If you care about them, you want to be supportive. However, some types of support could actually make their symptoms worse, subtly encouraging them to remain on their current trajectory. This helps no one.

How to Stop Enabling Individuals with Borderline Personality Disorder

It is important to reward healthy behaviors and be careful not to reinforce unhealthy ones. Some healthy BPD behaviors that should be supported include:

- those aimed at achieving independence and autonomy
- self-care
- self-improvement, including education and medical treatment
- uplifting others
- courtesy
- responding positively to others
- being responsible
- being respectful (Lobel, 2020)

Rewards can be verbal validations, such as affirming that what they just did for someone was positive or that you are enjoying being with them.

Don't reward unhealthy behaviors. Avoid giving in, no matter how much they try to manipulate, threaten, or cajole you. Doing so enables these behaviors and may worsen their disorder in the long term. This isn't easy. You might be tempted to give in if the conflict escalates or if you don't understand how rewarding their unhealthy behavior prevents them from healing. If they threaten to self-harm, establish whether they are serious and get professional help immediately if they are.

Practical Steps

There are several things you can do to encourage individuals with BPS to enter treatment if they have not already done so. Some examples are listed below:

- If you are providing financial support, this might be enabling them. Ensure that you know how they are going to use these funds.
- Don't fear conflict. If behaviors are hurtful or harmful to you or others, then speak to them about it—if you don't, then you are effectively enabling these behaviors. You can use validation techniques to minimize their negative reactions.
- Don't lie for them or cover up for them when they behave irresponsibly. They need to take responsibility for their own actions.
- Decide that any codependent aspects of your relationship with them need to stop. Shift your focus to other people or activities so you aren't constantly trying to please them. This might automatically reduce your enabling behavior.
- Become less helpful and set boundaries until they enter treatment. Reward them when they do so by looking

after things for them at home, taking care of their children, and so on.

- Don't tolerate their hurtful behaviors. Those close to people with BPD sometimes become inured to their behaviors and ignore them, even when those behaviors are hurtful or harmful. Never do this, even if the person refuses treatment (*Helping a Loved One With BPD*, 2011).

Practicing Mindfulness

Mindfulness is developing an awareness of things that are happening around us. This encourages deeper levels of change. Several studies have found that practicing mindfulness can literally change your brain, especially the parts involved in learning, memory, and processing emotion (Crumpler, 2022).

Meditation is often used to promote mindfulness. Sit alone in a quiet place where there are no distractions, including your phone. Close your eyes and breathe deeply. Let your thoughts come and go without judging them or feeling obliged to take action.

You don't need to meditate to be mindful. Doing gentle exercises or journaling will also help you identify and process your emotions.

Techniques for Beginners

Set aside time each day to develop mindfulness. Start with 30 minutes in the morning and ten minutes before bed (Crumpler, 2022). If your schedule is very busy, you can spend less time on this activity. Don't set a timeline for results, as everyone's journey is different, and pressuring yourself can impede your progress— there is no one-size-fits-all approach. Do mindfulness exercises regularly until it becomes a habit.

Exercises to Get You Started

Below are three easy techniques for beginners:

The 4-7-8 Breathing Technique

- Find a quiet, comfortable place and sit down.
- Exhale through your mouth.
- For four seconds, breathe in deeply through your nose and hold your breath for seven seconds.
- Exhale loudly for eight seconds out of your mouth.
- If this is difficult initially, you can work up to these numbers.

Body Scanning

In this technique, you will filter out the world's noise to establish your feelings and emotions.

- Lie down in a comfortable, quiet space, close your eyes, and relax.
- Focus on each part of your body, starting with your head.
- Pay attention to any sensations you feel and focus on these briefly.
- Let your thoughts drift as you move on to the next part of your body.
- Finish up with your toes.

Moving Mindfully

If you're going for a walk or jog, you can be mindful while you do this. Pay attention to your surroundings. What scents do you smell? What sounds do you hear? What do you see? How do you feel as your session continues?

By increasing your awareness of the world around you, you can start feeling calmer (Crumpler, 2022).

Interactive Element: Becoming Your Own Person

Have a pen and paper handy. Find a quiet place and consider your relationship with the individual with BPD in your life from all angles. Using the pointers mentioned in this chapter, establish whether there are any signs of codependency.

Ask yourself the following questions:

- When did you last do anything for yourself—just yourself?
- How could you make more time for yourself this week?
- How could you communicate with this person who needs to become more independent when you are not around?
- Phone an old friend who you always found supportive and rekindle that friendship.
- Practice mindfulness using a technique mentioned in this chapter.

Develop a strategy to help you address codependency issues and your own enabling behaviors. Use the skills you have learned throughout this book so far to assist you.

Key Takeaways

Codependency occurs when you become so focused on someone else's needs and desires that you neglect your own, and your personal growth becomes stunted. You might feel resentful at having to do so much for them at the expense of things you could do for yourself. People with BPD can also become codependent because of their extreme fear of abandonment. They might use several forms of coercion, including manipulation, control, and threats, to force you to meet their needs. You might become frustrated and exhausted because you have no time for yourself, and you could risk burning out. People with BPD who manipulate those closest to them to ensure that their own needs are met, regardless of other people's needs and desires, can also experience these feelings.

People with low self-esteem, insecure attachment styles, and those who rely on others for their sense of self-worth are more likely to become codependent. Being codependent is not being compassionate because your identity depends on the other person's world, as opposed to empathizing with their pain.

You may unwittingly encourage destructive behaviors by giving in to manipulation and controlling tactics rather than setting boundaries and rewarding positive behavior as opposed to detrimental behavior.

Some techniques for dealing with codependency include building self-esteem, recognizing your attachment style, finding time to be alone, improving communication, focusing on personal growth, and developing mindfulness.

In the next chapter, you will discover how to deal with the impact having a person with BPD in your life is likely to have on your mental health.

Chapter 6

Dealing With the Impact of BPD on Your Mental Health

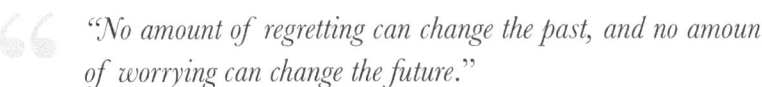 *"No amount of regretting can change the past, and no amount of worrying can change the future."*

— Roy T. Bennett

I n this chapter, you'll understand the effect being close to an individual with BPD can have on your mental health. You'll also discover strategies for prioritizing your self-care and incorporating these into your life.

Recognizing Signs of Trauma

Being close to someone who suffers from BPD can be extremely traumatic. You need to deal with the extreme highs and lows of their moods, as well as their abusive, manipulative, and controlling ways, not to mention changing your own responses to their behavior. Because these things are happening all the time, you may not realize the impact right away.

The extent of your distress might take some time to become apparent. Below are a few pointers to help you identify whether your relationship with an individual with BPD is becoming traumatic. You might notice that you:

- constantly feel anxious, "on edge," worried, or frightened
- feel hopeless, helpless, or depressed
- feel worthless or inadequate because you are not being treated with love and respect
- have flashbacks to traumatic events in which both of you were involved
- avoid certain situations or people who might trigger them
- feel guilty or responsible for the problems in the relationship
- have difficulty trusting the other person because you are always waiting for something negative to happen
- have difficulty regulating your emotions—you might be triggered more easily
- feel isolated
- feel emotionally or physically numb
- feel defensive
- be startled by the individual with BPD when they move unexpectedly
- feel irritable
- experience negative emotions
- have difficulty sleeping
- find it hard to focus on others
- avoid certain topics when you speak to them
- have negative feelings and beliefs about them
- be paranoid
- have nightmares or intrusive thoughts

- feel confused
- apologize continuously
- withdraw from other people who could support you (*10 Signs You're Experiencing Trauma*, 2023; Gillihan, 2023; Steber, 2021)

If you are experiencing several of the above symptoms and are in a relationship, then your best option would be to leave your partner with BPD. However, if you do not choose to or cannot leave the relationship because you are their parent, child, sibling, or any other close family member, then this chapter will provide you with some coping guidelines.

The Importance of Self-Care

If you are close to someone who has BPD, it's vital to prioritize self-care. To improve your relationship, you need to stop them from hurting you, as well as others who are close to them. Their ties to you can feel all-consuming, but it's important to develop your own support systems and have healthy outlets for your stress and emotions. You can't help someone develop good relationships if you yourself are overwhelmed.

Protecting your own physical safety and mental health by practicing self-care is a crucial priority. This will help to reduce stress, improve your immunity, and raise your energy.

It can be tempting to give your loved one with BPD every ounce of your time and energy, but finding time to be with encouraging, nurturing people is important because you also need support. Developing a life of your own will recharge your batteries while enabling you to relax and have fun. Everyone will benefit from taking a little time out. Joining a support group for families and friends of people with BPD might also be helpful, as participants share their experiences and insights with others having similar difficulties.

Both you and others who are close to your loved one with BPD need to take care of your physical health by eating properly, exercising sufficiently, and getting enough quality sleep. These things can easily be neglected when everyone gets caught up in the drama. Being in top physical form will improve your stress management as well.

Remaining calm when dealing with someone with BPD, so things don't spiral out of control, can be very taxing. There are ways to relieve the stress so you can be there for them without falling apart yourself.

10 Self-Care Ideas to Try

Here are ten great self-care activities that can give you and others on the receiving end a boost while taking a break:

Watching a Movie or Series Intentionally

Taking time out to watch a movie or series and deliberately removing your attention from your relationship can be a great way to decompress. This gives your brain a break. You can reset, so when you go back to dealing with the relationship, you'll feel refreshed.

Going Outside in Nature

When you're caught up in a difficult, demanding relationship, it's easy to forget how therapeutic it is to go outside and take in some natural beauty. If you can do this actively by hiking, walking, running, canoeing, or sailing, so much the better. Being in nature will automatically lift your mood, clear your thinking, sharpen your focus, and make you feel calmer. Outdoor time can also reduce stress hormones and generate feel-good ones, so you'll be more relaxed afterward.

Planting Something

Planting in a garden has significant benefits. Getting your hands dirty can literally make you happier and healthier, as soil contains feel-good microbes. Plus, you get vegetables, fruit, and flowers, all of which improve your quality of life.

Donating Your Time

Volunteering counters loneliness, raises self-esteem, relieves anxiety, and gives you a sense of purpose outside of your relationship.

Discovering a New Podcast

People's moods change in response to the tones of voices they hear, so plug into your favorite inspiring podcast for an instant boost. It can also make mundane chores go faster.

Planning a Getaway

Arranging a getaway is always fun, and it's an instant mood booster as you contemplate all the interesting things you might do. Whether you're discovering fresh places or revisiting old haunts, planning a trip is a great way to escape from reality. And you might actually take the vacation, too.

Taking a Course

It's always stimulating and exciting to learn new things, so list things you've always wanted to do—dancing, photography, flower arranging, a gourmet cooking course—and book your spot. Besides exercising your brain, you could make new friends.

Getting Creative

You don't have to be Picasso to draw or paint. Buy some adult coloring books and colored pencils, and you'll soon be absorbed. If you prefer knitting or sewing, channel your creative energies in this direction. You might add some new clothes or an attractive sweater to your wardrobe.

Call a Friend Who Makes You Laugh

Laughter is the best medicine, and medical research supports this (Krstic & Dolgoff, 2022). Social laughter releases feel-good hormones in our brains. Laughing together can strengthen your relationships with others (Krstic & Dolgoff, 2022).

Using Breathing Techniques

Breathing is a great way to relieve frustration and stress. It can quickly take the edge off after a tough day or when a loved one with BPD is having an episode.

Breath work refers to deep breathing that starts in your diaphragm, also known as belly breathing. Several breathing exercises can improve your physical, mental, and spiritual health. You can do breathwork without meditation. Breathing techniques help to relieve the following symptoms:

- stress, tension, anxiety, depression, and substance abuse
- post-traumatic stress disorder (PTSD)
- hypertension
- type 2 diabetes
- asthma symptoms

It boosts immunity and memory, promotes better sleep, and improves the quality of life for those living with serious illnesses. Deep breathing reduces your body's stress responses and creates calmness (Majsiak & Young, 2022).

Quick Tips for Beginners

- Start slowly and do only one minute of deep breathing (Majsiak & Young, 2022).
- Focus on breathing from your lower abdomen and use your hand so you can feel it moving.
- Breath work oxygenates the brain, releasing carbon dioxide, so it's a natural process.
- Find a technique that works for you.

Breath Work—A How-To Guide

The exercises detailed here focus on slow, deep breathing using your diaphragm.

Diaphragm Breathing

1. Sit up or lie down on your back.
2. Rest your hands on your belly just below your navel. Breathe in, feeling your belly soften and expand and shrink toward your spine as you exhale.

3. Place one hand on your ribs and the other on your belly. Feel your lungs expand and your belly soften as you inhale.
4. Move your rib hand to just below the collarbone. Inhale, feeling your belly soften, your ribs expand, and your upper chest enlarge. Exhale, letting everything go.
5. Do 5–10 repetitions in the morning and again in the evening before bed. You can do these exercises whenever you feel stressed.

Alternate Nostril Yoga Breathing

1. Sit comfortably, resting one hand on your knee. Gently close your left nostril with your left thumb and inhale slowly. Remove your finger from your left nostril and close your right nostril with your ring finger.
2. Hold your breath for a moment before exhaling through your left nostril.
3. Inhale through the now-open left nostril. Holding your breath, take your ring finger off the right nostril and close your left nostril with your left thumb once again. Exhale through the right nostril.
4. Repeat 5–10 times through both nostrils.

Ocean Sounding Breath

Do this exercise while sitting upright.

1. Take a deep breath through your nose.
2. Exhale slowly, making a gentle "haaa" ocean sound. If you're a beginner, you can open your mouth. As you become more proficient, you can exhale without opening your mouth.

3. Repeat until you feel relaxed.

Buteyko Breathing Technique

This is helpful if you're hyperventilating.

1. Sit down, elongating your spine and staying upright.
2. You will only breathe through your nose. Take some deep breaths to start off with.
3. After a relaxing exhale, hold your breath and gently plug your nose. This is the control pause.
4. Wait until your body shows that you need to breathe. Gently release your nose and inhale slowly and naturally. If your diaphragm moves involuntarily, don't panic.
5. Breathe normally again for at least ten seconds.
6. Repeat 3–5 times.

Laughter Yoga

1. Stand up, smile, and stand with your hands on your hips. Inhale, cross your right hand over to meet your left, and clap your hands, exhaling, "Ho, ho."
2. Then, raise your arms diagonally so your hands are on the right side of your head and clap, exhaling and saying, "Ha, ha, ha."
3. Repeat this three times. After the last "Ha, ha, ha," reach both arms above your head, shout "Yay!" and start laughing.

Heart Rate Variability Biofeedback

You might work with a biofeedback specialist when you do this breathing exercise, which means you'll be hooked up to monitors.

You can do this at home, but you need to measure your heart rate. You can use an app or a smartwatch.

1. Sit down and relax.
2. Using your device monitor, note your current heart rate.
3. Breathe deeply into your belly, imagining that you are on a rollercoaster. When you inhale, the car goes up the track, and when you exhale, it's going down. Do this smoothly, pausing between each inhale and exhale.
4. After five breaths, check your heart rate. The idea is to get your heart rate below what it was when you began.
5. Once you reach your goal, this exercise is completed.

Staying Healthy

It's important not to let your health regimen slide when coping with an individual with BPD. Staying healthy will help you cope with stress, together with their mental and emotional demands.

Exercise

Do physical activity every day, such as walking or cycling to work, doing household chores, gardening, or work-related activities. You can also enjoy active leisure pursuits like hiking, walking, running, dancing, swimming, or taking part in sports. While physical activity is often undertaken to lose weight, increase muscularity, and improve flexibility when you are involved with a loved one with BPD, you may derive several mental health benefits, some of which are listed below:

- Research shows that physical activity can lift one's mood. After exercising, study participants became calmer, mentally sharper, and happier. The benefits were greatest when participants felt depressed beforehand. Low-intensity aerobic exercise conducted for 30 minutes 3–5 times a week was found to be best for generating positive results.

- When you are stressed, your body experiences physiological changes, which can make you more emotional. Signs of stress usually include sleeping difficulties, loss of appetite, and excessive sweating. When you are stressed, your body releases hormones that raise your blood pressure, increase your heart rate, and inhibit digestion. Cortisol, a stress hormone, releases carbohydrates and fats into the bloodstream to generate more energy.

- Exercise generates improved self-esteem and feelings of self-worth, which influence how we cope with stress. This is effective for everyone, regardless of age or gender.

- Getting regular exercise relieves depression. It also reduces mild anxiety and can be helpful for those diagnosed with an anxiety disorder. Physical activity costs little and can be done almost anywhere (Mental Health Foundation, 2022).

Healthy Eating

Getting optimal nutrition maintains your energy levels, regulates your moods, and helps you cope with stress. Healthy eating means eating fresh vegetables and fruit, protein, whole grains, and dairy products. Choose low-fat or fat-free dairy options or use alternatives like soy or lactose-free milk if you have problems with lactose. Protein can be obtained from seafood, lean meat, poultry, eggs, legumes (peas, beans, and lentils), soy, nuts, and seeds.

Getting Enough Fiber

Increasing the fiber in your diet helps control blood sugar and reduce high cholesterol, as well as maintaining digestive health. Fresh fruits and vegetables, together with whole grains, nuts, seeds, and legumes, are all good fiber sources. Incorporate more of these into your diet by slicing up fresh vegetables to eat as snacks, having oatmeal or whole grain cereal for breakfast, adding beans or lentils to salads, and enjoying fruit with a meal or as a dessert.

Adding Minerals and Vitamins

Calcium and vitamin D together are essential for bone health. Drinking a fortified drink or taking supplements are the best ways to ensure that you receive enough. Eat a can of sardines or salmon that contains bones every week. Bok choy, collard greens, mushrooms, spinach, and taro root are good plant-based sources of these nutrients.

Potassium benefits your kidneys, heart, muscles, and nerves. Having insufficient potassium increases blood pressure, reduces the calcium in your bones, and increases the risk of developing kidney stones. Beet greens, lima beans, and Swiss chard are good sources. Drinking orange, pomegranate, or prune juice and eating bananas will all add potassium to your diet.

Reducing Added Sugar

Many processed foods and beverages contain added sugar. This can lead to weight gain, type 2 diabetes, and heart disease. Here are a few tips to avoid consuming hidden sugars:

- Drink water instead of sweetened beverages, using fruit slices or herbs to add flavor.
- Add fruit or berries to cereals and yogurt for sweetness.

- Avoid buying sugary drinks and snacks, and purchase vegetables, fruit, nuts, and seeds instead.
- Avoid adding whipped cream and flavorings at coffee shops.
- Choose foods with less added sugar—this will be indicated on product labels (CDC, 2022).

Avoiding Saturated Fats

Some dietary fat is essential for optimal health and proper functioning of the body. Saturated fats occur in fatty meats, butter, cream, full-fat cheese, sausages, and whole milk. Replace these with unsaturated fats. For example, you could use low-fat yogurt and an avocado to make your morning smoothie instead of whole milk. Sprinkle nuts and seeds over salads and other foods instead of cheese. Eat beans or seafood instead of fatty meats for protein. Eat low-fat cheeses and drink low-fat milk.

Reduce Sodium

Eating too much salt can put you at risk for high blood pressure, heart attacks, and strokes. Nearly all the sodium consumed in America is in processed foods. When cooking, use lemon juice, salt-free spice blends, and herbs to flavor foods. Look for low-sodium options when shopping for food, and buy unprocessed foods that you can cook at home.

Having a Colorful Plate

Aim for having a variety of colors on your plate to ensure that you're receiving plenty of vitamins, minerals, and beneficial compounds.

Getting Enough Sleep

Many of us are sleep-deprived. Working long hours and trying to find time to enjoy leisure activities or spend time with loved ones often makes it hard to get enough sleep. Using technology also makes it more difficult to fall asleep. Below are a few tips for getting better sleep:

- Avoid having any electronic devices, including a television and your phone, in your bedroom.
- Make sure that you go to bed and wake at the same time each day, even on weekends.
- Don't eat a large meal or drink caffeinated or alcoholic beverages before bedtime.
- Your bedroom should be dark, quiet, at a comfortable temperature, and have a relaxed atmosphere.
- Exercise. Being physically active during the day can make it easier to fall asleep at night (CDC, 2022).

Interactive Element: Prioritizing Yourself

Finding time for self-care can be difficult, especially when a loved one with BPD is demanding, but it's essential to look after yourself. This will help you stay calm and relaxed and be more mentally alert. Ignoring your own physical and mental needs will make it much harder to cope with stress, causing stress-related illnesses or burnout.

Get out your diary or the calendar app on your phone and schedule daily exercise, as well as mindful breathing or meditation. If they see you are doing this, it might inspire them, too.

Discuss with them your need for "me" time. Think about activities you enjoy—or choose two or three activities from the ones mentioned in this chapter—and decide when you are going to take time out. Book a course, make that phone call, schedule a movie night, or arrange that day hike you've been wanting to do.

Think about your eating habits and decide whether you need to change your shopping and eating routines to ensure that you are eating a more balanced diet. If you are living with a loved one with BPD, then discuss this with them when they are calm, explaining that this will also benefit them. Poor eating habits can exacerbate low moods.

If you are struggling to get quality sleep, follow the guidelines in this chapter and see if things improve.

Key Takeaways

Dealing with the demands of a relationship with someone with BPD can take its toll on your mental and physical health. To endure the intense mood swings, abuse, and threats, you will need to ensure that you care for yourself so that you can cope.

There are several deep breathing exercises you can do to relieve stress. Do them once or twice a day, or while the individual with BPD is experiencing an episode, to keep you calm and focused. It's important to schedule "me" time to give you a break and enable you to be yourself without worrying about someone else's problems. There are several activities you can do to relax, connect with other people, and expand your horizons.

Being physically active every day is a proven stress reliever and releases feel-good hormones that will boost your mood. You'll be more relaxed and cope better. Ensure that you get proper nutrition to help you cope with stress, keep your mind sharp, and prevent you from succumbing to your loved one's emotional and mental demands. Finally, make sure you get enough quality sleep so you function at your best, whether at work or play or when dealing with your relationship.

Your loved one is likely in therapy or is considering it, but it's possible that you might need to talk to a professional, too. Not everyone will appreciate what you are going through. Therapy can provide you with an independent sounding board and enable you to cope with your partner's erratic behavior.

Chapter 7

Therapeutic Approaches and Their Efficacy

 "If you are broken, you do not have to stay broken."

— Selena Gomez

This chapter discusses the efficacy of different therapies and treatment options. Here, you can also discover strategies to employ if your partner with BPD refuses to seek help.

Treatment Options for Borderline Personality Disorder

The main treatment for BPD is psychotherapy, also known as talk therapy. This aims to teach individuals with BPD techniques and skills for managing their thoughts and emotions. There are different types of psychotherapy that are specifically used to treat BPD, each one of which has different methods. This is not a blanket approach—sometimes, an individual needs to try more than one type of therapy until they find one that works for them.

In this section, you'll find out about the different types of therapy available to people with BPD and what each one involves.

Dialectical Behavior Therapy

Developed by clinical psychologist Dr. Marsha Linehan, Dialectical Behavior Therapy (DBT) was one of the first psychotherapies found to be effective for people suffering from BPD. As mentioned previously, DBT is a form of cognitive behavior therapy that reveals the thoughts and beliefs that underpin behaviors and actions typical of BPD. Mindfulness is an important component of DBT. Individuals learn skills to help them cope with powerful emotions and manage stress. DBT is the most effective therapy for BPD, as it helps such individuals stay in treatment, as well as reducing self-harm and hospitalization.

Schema-Focused Therapy

This form of therapy combines aspects of cognitive behavior therapy and other psychoanalytic theories. It is based on the idea that unmet childhood needs can cause those with BPD to have a distorted, unhealthy view of themselves and the world. Schema-focused therapy works to change these maladaptive beliefs and behaviors, replacing them with healthier thoughts and ways of coping.

Transference-Focused Psychotherapy

Studies conducted on transference-focused therapy (TFP) show that it may be as or more effective than DBT (Salters-Pedneault, 2020). At the heart of this therapy is transference, when the feelings and expectations present in the client's earliest relationships are transferred to someone with whom they are currently interacting. This is an important concept in psychodynamic therapy. TFP uses the relationship the client has with the therapist to determine how the client relates to others. The therapist then uses this knowledge to help the client become more effective in their other relationships.

Mentalization-Based Therapy

Mentalization-Based Therapy (MBT) is another form of psychotherapy that has been researched to determine its effectiveness for BPD. It is believed that it could ease depression and anxiety in people with BPD and may also improve social functioning. The process works by helping the client recognize different mental states, including their own feelings and thoughts, as well as those of others. Being able to do this enables them to see how their thoughts contribute to their behavior.

Systems Training for Emotional Predictability and Problem Solving

Systems Training for Emotional Predictability and Problem Solving (STEPPS) is a skills-based group program conducted alongside other therapies. STEPPS defines BPD as an "emotional intensity disorder" and assists sufferers with regulating their behavior and emotions. It also helps those in a BPD support group, including friends and family members, to understand the disorder. The idea is to enable individuals with BPD to form healthy relationships with those tasked with reinforcing these new skills. STEPPS also teaches self-care, including improving sleeping patterns and healthy eating, as well as ways of avoiding self-harm. Both STEPPS and DBT were found effective in significantly reducing BPD symptoms within six months, although

DBT had a more positive effect on modulating behavioral symptoms (Eagle, 2020).

Self-Help

Self-help strategies should be included in any BPD treatment program. They should supplement therapy and not be used on their own. People with BPD should be encouraged to learn as much as possible about their disorder, find positive ways to express and regulate their emotions, and learn healthy coping skills.

Self-Care Strategies for Individuals with Borderline Personality Disorder

- Hit a pillow, do vigorous exercise, listen to loud music, do some deep cleaning, or garden when feeling angry, frustrated, or restless.
- Listen to uplifting music, write a comforting letter to yourself, or watch a favorite TV show or film to counter feelings of sadness or depression.
- When feeling tense or anxious, people with BPD can enjoy a warm shower or take ten deep breaths and count them out loud. They can also practice some of the breathing exercises referred to in chapter six.
- Chew something strong-tasting like chili or ginger, suck on sour candy, drink iced water, or clap. Noticing the sensations these create in the body could help to dispel feelings of disassociation (Eagle, 2020).

Medication

While there are no approved medications for treating BPD, the following may be prescribed by doctors or psychiatrists:

- Antidepressants or antianxiety medication can help to ease anxiety and depression. However, some are addictive and should be used with caution.
- Antipsychotics may help with BPD symptoms, such as anger, paranoia, and impulsiveness.
- Mood stabilizers could help to reduce extreme emotional reactions and impulsiveness (Salters-Pedneault, 2020).

Encouraging Therapy for Individuals with Borderline Personality Disorder

Many people with mental illness are in denial or simply do not realize the extent of the problem. This is often because of a lack of self-awareness or irrational thought patterns brought on by the disorder. Some people with BPD might reject their diagnosis because it is simply too unpalatable for them to accept. When families, friends, and partners reach out to their loved ones to seek treatment, they may be seen as the adversary.

For therapy to work, it is essential that your loved one with BPD want to get better. If they enter therapy because of your insistence or because they are afraid that you will abandon them if they don't, then this will not facilitate their treatment. Your loved one might also perceive your efforts as threatening or condescending. Even if they enter treatment, they may become resentful and passive-aggressive, which are forms of resistance.

Remember that you cannot force someone to get treatment. Don't feel guilty if your loved one refuses to be treated—you are not responsible for their decisions, although it can be hard for you to watch them having emotional meltdowns or be on the receiving end of their dysfunctional behaviors.

It's important to ensure that your loved one is motivated—they need to want to get well of their own volition, not just because you say so. This is also important for ensuring that they remain in treatment and continue to take any prescription medications. DBT is a very useful treatment because it has motivation built in.

To get them into therapy, it's important to validate them as much as possible. Making statements like, "You really should go," will make them feel judged, further demotivating them. A better approach would be to tell them how difficult going into therapy can be and how much you respect them for trying. You can also mention how hard it is to open up to someone you don't know and tell them all your deepest secrets. Keep planting seeds.

Tips for Talking About Therapy

This conversation can be tricky, and there is a lot vested in the outcome. Here are some suggestions for talking to your loved one about therapy:

- Show support and be careful to use language that doesn't stigmatize them. BPD was once considered a difficult, untreatable condition, and many people do not understand this disorder, which has made the diagnosis very stigmatizing. Assure them of your support throughout the process.
- Timing is important. Broach the subject when your loved one is calm, rational, and seems to be open to the

idea. Don't talk about therapy when they are in a bad mood, tired, or focused on something important, like a work deadline.

- Be sensitive to not only their emotional readiness to talk about getting help but also to where you have this conversation. Find a quiet, peaceful place where you cannot be overheard, as they will probably want some privacy. That way, they are likely to feel respected and in control (being in control is very important for people with BPD).
- Ensure that the conversation stays calm, friendly, and relaxed.
- Be prepared for resistance, and think about how you will make your case beforehand.

  - You could mention that your relationship with them is important and might improve if they seek therapy. Avoid giving them an ultimatum, as this will make them stressed and be counterproductive.
  - Focus on their positive qualities and remember to validate them.
  - Mention some areas of dysfunctional behavior you have been experiencing with them. This will make it more difficult for them to deny that there is a problem.

- Offer meaningful support. You could, for example, help them find a suitable therapist in the area based on their preferences, offer to look after their children while they are in therapy sessions, or drive them to evening group sessions. If they are uncomfortable, offer to sit in the waiting room during the first few visits (Jones, 2017).

Managing Expectations

There are many individuals with BPD who desperately want to get their lives on track, especially as they age and realize that the behaviors that served them so well during their dysfunctional childhood are no longer appropriate. BPD never completely heals, but if the individual is prepared to work closely with the therapist, then they have a good chance of going into remission. Remission improves the longer the sufferer can stay in therapy, with symptoms reducing by as much as 40%–50% within two years (Choi-Kain & Gunderson, 2009).

Forms of Resistance

Even if an individual with BPD agrees to therapy, they often interfere with the treatment process. If there are problems with heightened emotional reactions or a history of self-harming, these need to be attended to first. Very often, individuals with BPD do not respond to regular psychological treatment, and the medications prescribed for allied anxiety or mood disorders are ineffective. DBT and schema-based therapy were specifically developed to manage this.

Acting out by self-harming or other attention-getting behaviors is another way individuals with BPD avoid talking about their feelings. This is also a form of resistance. Sometimes, they may refuse to discuss family difficulties with the therapist, and therapy may be ended by the family, who fear exposure.

Even if the individual with BPD enters treatment, there is no guarantee that they will stick with it. Some reasons include their fluctuating sense of self, which interferes with their goals and motivations for getting better. Sometimes, they feel nothing will help, and they cannot change.

Others drop out because working on yourself can be extremely difficult. Sometimes, the therapist will inadvertently trigger a person's defensive behaviors because they cannot cope with the level of emotion that washes over them. They may leave therapy rather than confront their problems. Therapists who might become or replace the BPD's favorite person, especially during transference, may find themselves on the receiving end of bizarre behavior. Another difficulty is that BPD often presents with other disorders, such as anxiety disorder. A sufferer with debilitating social anxiety may be too afraid to leave home to attend DBT group therapy, for example.

Some people with BPD are also challenged by therapists who have an insufficient understanding of BPD and lack compassion, becoming critical and patronizing. It is essential that therapists create a safe space where individuals with BPD can express their pain. Therapists need to absorb the anger or other negative responses this generates without reacting. Your loved one with BPD is not lashing out at the therapist personally but expressing their pain to someone who may enable them to make sense of it.

Many people with BPD drop out of therapy because of the sheer difficulty of confronting themselves and their problems. However, for those who stick with it, it is possible to change their thoughts, emotions, and behaviors. (Choi-Kain & Gunderson, 2009 Borderline Personality Disorder and Resistance to Treatment).

Success Stories

Christina has been working on her BPD since 2015. She has found mindfulness helpful in coping with her fear of abandonment. She has built three good, stable friendships but is avoiding romantic relationships because of her tendency to idolize her partner, which causes her to behave irrationally. She has learned to argue without devaluing others. She has a much stronger sense of self. When this wavers, she does something productive and then sleeps on it. She is less impulsive. She no longer idealizes suicide but practices gratitude instead. Mindfulness also helps with her mood swings—she still struggles in this area. When her father died, she experienced intense feelings of emptiness but could work through them with her therapist. She still struggles with tremendous anger, although it is no longer explosive and does not last long. She occasionally experiences paranoia, but only for a short while. She has less depression and suicidal thoughts.

Mike is a therapist working with people with BPD. For individuals with BPD to change, they need to be motivated. Many come to therapy and just pretend to get help. Others stay motivated because they have a crisis, but their focus wanes once the difficulty is resolved. Asking individuals with BPD to control their emotions is setting them up for a future explosion—it's more constructive for them to reframe their emotions. Mike helps them take responsibility for their own lives. He and his clients work together to find which therapy works best. There are setbacks, and sometimes, individuals with BPD need medication. Once their inner abandoned, neglected child is dealt with, there is immediate relief. They no longer need to be hypervigilant and feel calm and relaxed. People with BPD then learn that they can choose their emotions and responses. They discover they are valuable human beings. Once they resolve this, many people with BPD report feeling truly alive for the first time. They also learn important life skills, like setting boundaries, managing their triggers and thoughts, doing meditation, and tracking their progress. Many of Mike's clients stop wanting to die, avoid abusive relationships, renew relationships with their parents after years of being estranged, and can bless their own children.

Interactive Element: Choosing the Right Treatment

Read over the chapter and answer the following questions to help you improve your current situation:

- How has your loved one been doing lately? Have they decided to get treatment?
- If not, how could you start a conversation with them to encourage them to try therapy, as well as other treatments such as mindfulness?
- How would you discuss the different treatment options with them?
- How could you support them when they go into therapy?
- If they are receiving treatment, have you noticed any improvement with the current treatment? If not, how could you talk to them about changing to a different therapy?

Key Takeaways

There are several treatment options for BPD. The most often used and successful one is DBT. Other treatments include schema-focused therapy, MBT, STEPPS, and transference-focused therapy. These are often used with self-help actions like eating properly, getting enough exercise, and improving sleep patterns. As each individual with BPD is different, it's sometimes necessary to try different forms of treatment before establishing which one is the most effective. Medication can prevent wild mood swings and ease anxiety and depression.

Getting a loved one who has BPD into therapy is difficult, as they are inclined to resist the process, believing that there is nothing wrong with them. You cannot force them into therapy, and it will also be less effective if they feel coerced. When encouraging your loved one to undergo therapy, it's important to speak to them when they are in the right frame of mind and to offer them privacy. Ensure that you use validating statements explaining why you are having this conversation. Offer them support if they choose to go into therapy.

Being in therapy can be challenging, and many people with BPD drop out for various reasons. Therapists who do not understand BPD can also be judgmental and condescending. However, there are many positive stories of people who have persevered with therapy and have gone into remission, where their symptoms are reduced, and they can live normal lives.

In the next chapter, you'll discover more about how to find support for your loved one from both professionals and support groups.

Chapter 8

Seeking Support from Groups to Professionals

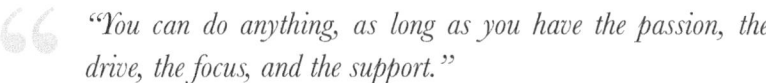

"You can do anything, as long as you have the passion, the drive, the focus, and the support."

— Sabrina Bryan

I f you are the partner, friend, or family member of someone with BPD, you may experience challenges and need to secure your own mental health. In this chapter, you'll discover groups, organizations, and professionals you can approach to develop your own support networks.

The Benefits of Support Groups

If you are in a relationship with a loved one with BPD, you will realize that it is a very complex mental illness with many facets. This can make it difficult to know how best to support them and aid in their recovery while also taking care of yourself.

Because so little is known about BPD, sufferers and their care-givers often experience negative reactions from others, which can be very isolating. As a result, many of those living with an individual with BPD find themselves with dwindling social outlets and little time to attend to their own social or personal needs. Support groups can help those involved with people who have BPD to become more self-assured, develop skills that make positive interactions more likely, and be better able to take care of their own mental and physical health.

Improving Communication Skills

Taking part in a BPD support group can improve how caregivers interact with institutions like schools, mental health organizations, and health insurance companies. Participants also learn how to have difficult discussions with their loved ones. This may not come easily, and support groups provide encouragement and empathy. They also focus on achieving radical acceptance. This means that they understand that the extreme behavior shown by someone with a BPD diagnosis is not manipulation but a way of ensuring that their deep-seated needs are met. Caregivers also learn to recognize the emotion behind their loved one's impulsive decisions.

Communication guidelines might look like this:

- Accept the person but not their behavior—you can voice your disagreement when necessary.
- If you are in a family situation, remember to spend time with other family members, especially other children.
- Choose your battles carefully.
- Take care of yourself so that you don't become unusually negative. Include activities you find enjoyable

and emotionally or physically fulfilling in your routine, as well as looking after your own physical health (O'Dougherty, 2021).

Being Part of a Community

Having a support group helps parents, spouses, and caregivers navigate these types of decisions and even find humor in their situations. Attending regular meetings, either in-person or through online video chat platforms, enables those caring for someone with BPD to join a community of people with similar experiences. This not only creates opportunities to be heard and understood but also provides practical advice and reminds caregivers to look after themselves as well.

Types of Support

Peer programs provide support and information for parents, partners, families, friends, and others in a relationship with someone with BPD. These may take the form of online or offline workshops or information sessions, where caregivers learn more about BPD, how to communicate effectively, and how to practice self-care. You can find out what to expect as a caregiver, as well as receive information about government resources that might be of help. There are also support groups tailored for families and young people.

Seeking Support for Yourself

As mentioned previously, caring for someone close to you who has BPD can be difficult. It can sap your energy and affect your own mental health, especially when leaving is not an option. You might find it difficult to talk to others about your feelings, especially if you are worn down by dealing with powerful emotions, needing to curb your loved one's impulsivity, or visiting emergency rooms when they are self-harming or suicidal. Being available 24/7 without respite can also take its toll.

Although the stigma against those with mental health issues is waning, you might still feel that you will be stigmatized if you wish to receive professional help. Doing so can be daunting, and you might not know how to go about it or whether you even need help at all. (Lovell 2022)

Benefits of Seeking Help

There are many advantages to joining support groups or entering therapy yourself when supporting a loved one with BPD.

- You will be less isolated in your struggle, as you will meet like-minded people who understand what you are experiencing and can help you talk through your emotions. Even if you opt for one-on-one therapy, your therapist is a nonjudgmental sounding board, providing you with tools to better manage the situation.
- Support groups and counseling can help you communicate better with not only the person with BPD in your life but your other loved ones, too. You will learn how to communicate clearly and honestly, building better, healthier relationships.
- Poor mental health often manifests in your physical health as well. It can affect things like sleep quality and eating patterns, as well as suppress your immune system.
- Receiving professional help will improve your coping skills and help you develop better strategies to work with your loved one. You will become more confident as you

navigate challenging and difficult situations with greater awareness.

- Mental health difficulties are often implicated in poor work performance, as they can reduce your motivation and make you feel negative and despondent. Talking about the difficulties you are experiencing as the caregiver of someone with BPD may improve your work performance, enabling you to work well even when you are under pressure at home.

- Finally, the skills you will learn during therapy will likely remain with you for life, making you a stronger person who is better able to cope with the difficulties of daily life, reduce stress, and know your limitations. The result will be a healthier, happier you.

When to Seek Professional Help

Perhaps you've been navigating the troubled waters of caring for your BPD loved one for so long that you're missing important signs that you need to get support. Indications that you need to seek help include:

- reduced concentration, especially at work
- friends and family voicing concerns about your mental health
- losing interest in things that once energized and excited you
- sleeping poorly
- being physically ill and experiencing a range of ailments, from stomach complaints to coughs and colds
- feeling isolated and alone
- having experienced a traumatic event

- abusing substances or changing your eating habits to cope (Perry, 2021)

It's important to reach out if you are feeling overwhelmed and noticing any of these signs of distress. Find a trained professional to talk to or join a support group to receive effective guidance and support.

Talking to Others

Given the stigma attached to BPD, you might find the suggestion of talking to others counterintuitive, but it can relieve the isolation and loneliness you might feel if you are caring for someone with BPD. If you have been able to keep at least part of your social network despite the difficulties, regularly reach out to caring, supportive, and nurturing friends.

Having an open, honest discussion with someone else about the difficulties you are experiencing may help to improve your mental health. Talking to someone who is not directly involved in your situation can enable you to get diverse perspectives and validation, develop coping strategies, and feel emotionally supported.

Talking to others will help you relieve stress, feel less isolated, and deepen your existing friendships. Getting another perspective might also help you make the right decisions concerning the person with BPD in your life, enabling you to express your thoughts and feelings without fearing judgment. Your friends might offer solutions or ideas that had not occurred to you. Being able to talk to someone can also make you more resilient.

Because caring for someone who has BPD can be very intense and sometimes traumatic, you might wonder who you can talk to besides a therapist. Start by making a list of all your social connections, including people you might not have spoken to for a while, people you've met on social media, extended family members, and co-workers.

Look at your list and consider which people have been empathetic in the past. Reach out to them and invite them out for a coffee. If you are working outside the home, meet them during your lunch break rather than after work. You might need to start slowly with newer friends as you build trust and get to know one another, but you could find someone with whom you can speak about your difficulties. Although your caregiving might seem all-consuming, remember to consider how you can provide support for your friends as well.

Another strategy is to visit a place of worship that reflects your spiritual or religious leanings and try to attend regularly. Places of worship often generate social connections with caring individuals, and it's highly likely that you can receive the support you need besides that provided by your BPD support group. If you cannot meet people in person, try connecting through social media or messaging apps.

Resources for Caregivers

In this section, you will find details of resources available for those who are caring for people with BPD.

Information and Support Groups

Natural Education Alliance for Borderline Personality Disorder

The Natural Education Alliance for Borderline Personality Disorder (NEABPD) offers a free, 8- or 12-week Family Connections course. Sessions are conducted weekly. The course can also be done as a 2-day or 4-day weekend option. This course educates, trains, and supports those caring for people with BPD or those who have emotional dysregulation (ED). The course is available in the United States, Canada, and Australia, with affiliates in other countries. Participants must be at least 18 years of age (NEABPD, 2011).

The Sashbear Foundation

This is the Canadian arm of NEABPD and provides courses in English and French. Training is given by family members of people with BPD, many of whom have experienced the same struggles as you. Courses and support groups are also available online.

National Alliance on Mental Illness Family Support Group

The National Alliance on Mental Illness (NAMI) offers peer-led support groups for those caring for people with mental illnesses. You will network with people who are experiencing the same difficulties as you and gain support from them. The groups are free and may meet weekly, biweekly, or monthly, depending on your location. Group sessions are between 60 and 90 minutes long, and all discussions are confidential. Visit the NAMI website to find a group near you or consider starting one if nothing is available (*BPD Family Communities*, 2015).

BPD Family

This is a message board and forum for people with BPD and their caregivers. Follow community guidelines when joining to get important information about BPD, ask questions, and receive help and advice from both professionals and lay people who are supporting people with BPD.

Helpful Books

Below are a few books you might find helpful:

- *Borderline Personality Disorder in Adolescents* by Blaise Aguirre
- *Borderline Personality Disorder Demystified* by Robert O. Friedel
- *Understanding and Treating Borderline Personality Disorder* by John H. Gunderson and Perry D. Hoffman
- *Savvy: Communication Skills for Family Members and Friends of Someone with Borderline Personality Disorder* by Karyn Hall
- *Borderline Personality Disorder Survival Guide* by Alexander Chapman and Kim Gratz
- *DBT for Dummies* by Gillian Galen & Blaise Aguirre
- *Mindfulness and Meditation: Your Questions Answered* by Blaise Aguirre
- *Building a Life Worth Living* by Marsha M. Linehan
- *Beyond Borderline-True Stories of Recovery* by John Gunderson and Perry Hoffman
- *Talking About BPD: A Stigma-Free Guide to Living a Calmer, Happier Life with Borderline Personality Disorder* by Kimberley Wilson

Interactive Element: Getting Much-Needed Support

You are not alone! There are many people who have someone with BPD in their lives and are experiencing the same challenges as you. It's essential to find ways in which you can be heard and supported as you navigate the difficulties and stresses connected with BPD. Just talking to other understanding people can make you feel less isolated. It can be especially helpful to join a support group with others in the same situation so you can share information, stories, and strategies from personal experience.

Below are a few questions to assist you in identifying potential support networks that may already exist in your work and social circles.

1. Do you feel you are supported at the moment, and to what extent?
2. When you need to talk, who do you turn to? List their names.
3. Can you think of other support networks that could help you feel less isolated?
4. How can you approach them and incorporate them into your life?
5. Which of the support options mentioned in this chapter could you contact?

Key Takeaways

Because relationships with people with BPD can be so intense, finding support is essential to protect your own mental health. You may be subject to verbal or physical abuse, the BPD relationship cycle, or the trauma of watching your loved one self-harm or attempt suicide. Fortunately, support groups, courses, and therapies are available.

Mental health support groups for those caring for individuals with BPD will enable you to interact with people who are experiencing the same things. Many are run by organizations that can provide more information about BPD and coping strategies. This will improve your communication skills and help you feel more connected, as well as provide you with resources. You can do online and offline courses and read books to help you navigate your loved one's BPD.

If you are experiencing mental health difficulties yourself, it is advisable to find a therapist who can help you develop better coping strategies and reduce stress. Remember to reach out to other friends and colleagues, as this will extend your support network.

If your partner or spouse is diagnosed with BPD, you may reach a point where you are considering whether to continue on or end the relationship. In the next chapter, you'll find guidelines for doing this, as well as advice on how to untangle yourself from your partner.

Chapter 9

Navigating Breakups and Letting Go

 "It is so hard to leave—until you leave.

And then it is the easiest goddamned thing in the world."

—John Green

It's all too much. You can no longer cope with the emotional rollercoaster, BPD relationship cycle, abuse, suicidal threats, and emergency room visits. You might need to cut ties to safeguard your own mental and physical health. Breaking up is hard to do, and it can be especially complicated if the other person has BPD. In this chapter, you'll find some guidelines to help you navigate this process.

Until Borderline Personality Disorder, Do Us Part

You realize that your relationship isn't a healthy one. You feel you've lost your way, and you're falling apart. You've done everything you can to appease and assist your partner with BPD, but it's not working. Perhaps you're attending a support group, and you've carved a bit of personal space. Good friends and family members might urge you to leave.

You keep focusing on the good times when your loved one is enthusiastic, excited, and obviously delighted to be with you. Maybe you're thrilled to be their favorite person, or they've brought out the Good Samaritan in you. You've decided that the problems are your fault, and you're determined to work through them. You might hold on to things they said when you first met, and you're hoping that love will conquer all. Perhaps you've seen all the facets of your relationship, and you feel you need to stay to help them, hold them together, and prevent them from going over the edge. You might have mentioned that you can't take it anymore, and they switch to being nice or become unusually clingy, making you have second thoughts. You might think that your relationship has turned a corner, but they've just ratcheted the relationship cycle up a notch. In fact, this might not be the first time you've considered leaving.

Things to Consider Before Leaving

Deciding to leave a relationship can be agonizing. There are a few things to consider before you tell them it's finally, irrevocably over.

When you're in a relationship with someone with BPD, no matter what type of relationship it is, the focus is usually on them. Think about yourself for a minute. How do *you* feel? Because of the nature of the disorder, many of those in relationships with someone with BPD feel alone and isolated. This gets worse over time because most people outside of the relationship don't understand BPD and how it manifests. You might feel stressed and uncertain. Perhaps the emotional turbulence, lying, and unfaithfulness have destroyed your trust. If they self-harm or have attempted suicide, you might be traumatized, anxious, or frightened.

If you are a partner or spouse, you might take on their household chores or care for their children when they are too fraught to do so. They might not work, so you're the breadwinner, too. All these additional responsibilities place an enormous burden on you, and you might feel tired and frustrated.

As mentioned previously, especially if you are married to someone with BPD, you are their partner, not their therapist. You are not their full-time caregiver, although it's easy to slip into that role. It's natural for you to want an emotional connection with your loved one. This might influence your decision to leave.

Options Before Leaving

If you'd like to have one last-ditch attempt to save the situation, try the following:

- You can go for counseling or therapy, which might help you cope better and decide whether leaving is the best option, as well as how to do this effectively.
- Discuss your feelings with your partner. This might encourage them to seek treatment if they are not already doing so and help them manage their symptoms better.
- Consider an intervention by other family members or a professional. Might this help to motivate the loved one with BPD to enter or continue with their treatment? (Robb-Dover, 2022)

Valid Reasons for Leaving

You might be vacillating between leaving and staying. Some of the key indicators that it's time to go include:

- Your loved one is engaging in risky behaviors like gambling, taking numerous lovers, reckless driving, substance abuse, and self-harming.
- Your loved one is refusing treatment, skipping therapy or group sessions, or not taking their medication.
- You are overwhelmed by additional responsibilities.
- You are the victim of physical threats and abuse.
- You are traumatized because of their repeated suicide attempts and self-harming (Robb-Dover, 2022).

Handling Breakups with Care and Sensitivity

Individuals with BPD have a heightened fear of abandonment, so breaking up requires careful thought and preparation. You might need to get guidance from a mental health professional. Be prepared for adversity and negativity. Ensure that you have a support structure in place—friends, family, or a support group that can help you navigate the transition. Arrange for a place to stay in case you need to remove yourself physically.

When breaking up with your partner, speak to them clearly and directly. Don't simply disappear or stop communicating with them, as this could trigger severe overreactions because of their fear of abandonment, and you don't want them to self-harm or hurt others. Avoid being critical or blaming; focus on your feelings and your decision to end the relationship. You don't need to justify your decision. You could even have this discussion in a neutral place with a close friend or trusted family member nearby to help if necessary.

Following the DBT method might help. This involves:

- being gentle and avoiding attacking, threatening, or guilt-tripping your partner
- acting interested, listening to their views without interrupting, and being sensitive to their feelings
- validating their feelings and problems without being judgmental
- being light-hearted and helping your partner process what is happening (*Breaking Up with Someone*, 2011)

It's vital to establish boundaries afterward, as your partner might want to reconnect, hoping to rekindle the relationship, which is part of the BPD relationship cycle. Stick to your decision and maintain your boundaries consistently. Be aware of your mental state, as leaving a BPD relationship can be emotionally draining and stressful. Process your emotions—with a therapist if necessary—and be sure to practice self-care.

Individuals with BPD might react extremely intensely and negatively once the reality of the breakup sets in. If they have a history of aggressive, violent behavior, take steps to ensure your safety. Ask friends and family to assist you, remain vigilant, and inform law enforcement if necessary.

If you need to engage with your former partner after your breakup, establish clear rules for these occasions. If personal communication is too stressful or emotional, you could use text messages or email. Keep your interactions brief and to the point. Avoid being drawn into arguments or discussions by reinforcing your boundaries.

You might need therapy to process your emotions after the breakup to become emotionally independent again. Therapy or counseling can help you deal with any lingering guilt, rebuild your self-esteem, and help you develop coping mechanisms, especially if you have experienced emotional or physical abuse.

Moving On and Letting Go

Letting go of your BPD relationship can be very difficult because these relationships have an addictive quality, especially if you've been experiencing the BPD relationship cycle. Feeling angry or upset after the breakup is normal and natural. Longing to have the relationship back is also common, especially when the relationship has been complex or toxic. When you feel this way, it's important to recall the unhealthy aspects of the relationship and why you ended it.

Allow yourself to feel your emotions. Bottling them up is a recipe for disaster. Talk to a trusted friend or therapist about your feelings, or write them down. The latter can be a helpful way to process emotions. Focus on the positives in your life and try not to dwell on the past. Holding onto the pain and hurt, constantly wondering what you could have done better, will prevent you from moving on and possibly finding a good, stable relationship.

Here are a few tips to help you stay focused:

- End communication altogether. This includes texts, emails, and social media. Block them if necessary.
- Delete all digital media concerning them and the relationship, such as photographs, videos, or memes, from your phone, laptop, and social media. Trash physical reminders like cards, framed photographs, and sentimental gifts. You need to move on.

- Fill your life with positivity, including things you might have neglected during your relationship. Take part in activities and hobbies you enjoy, sign up for a course, reconnect with friends, and spend time with family. This will make it easier to forget your ex.
- If you are struggling to move on, get professional help. Talking to a counselor or therapist can help you work through your feelings (Keen, 2022).

It can also be helpful to understand what happened and get closure. Reflect on the causes of your relationship's demise. Relationships with individuals with **BPD** can be extremely difficult, if not impossible, to maintain. If your ex was unwilling or unable to get help for their condition, the relationship was probably not going to succeed, anyway. You can talk to an understanding friend, a therapist, or a counselor to navigate your way back to emotional and mental health.

Surround yourself with supportive people who can help you through this difficult time. Find a support group of people who have been through a similar experience to provide you with a safe emotional space. Your relationship might have made you feel lonely and isolated, but connecting with others will help you become part of a community again.

It's vital to practice self-care after the breakup. Take care of your physical, mental, and emotional health. Exercise, eat properly, and make sure you get enough sleep. Give yourself time to grieve.

Quick Post-Breakup Tips for Borderline Personality Disorder Relationships

- Understand yourself and who you are. Focus on personal growth. This will improve your life and future relationships.
- Unpack your emotional baggage and ensure that you have eradicated unhealthy patterns before entering new relationships.
- Consider and try to understand your own role in the relationship so you don't make the same mistakes again. This will break the cycle.
- Learn to love yourself unconditionally. This is important and enables you to see the red flags in future relationships.
- Ending the relationship means that you can focus on yourself, enabling you to discover yourself, understand your situation, and learn how to develop healthy boundaries.
- Seeing a therapist may help you regain your personal identity, recognize codependent traits, and create healthy boundaries.(Thirahealth.com 2023)

Case Studies

Grace's Story: Tom is Not His Borderline Personality Disorder

Grace and Tom have been together for a year, and she recently moved in with him. She says it hasn't been easy, but he is her best friend and the love of her life. When he told her he suffers from BPD, she researched it and found that most of the information about individuals with BPD relates mainly to their symptoms. It was tempting to make assumptions, but her boyfriend had repeatedly proven her wrong.

They have had their share of ups and downs. He swings from idolizing her to devaluing her, treating her like a goddess one moment, and then focusing on all the negative aspects of her personality and being hypercritical. Sometimes, their relationship is all about his needs, and then it's all about hers. He takes full responsibility for his outbursts, is deeply hurt about what he says to her at those times, and apologizes afterward. These incidents frequently follow discussions they have about the deep, unresolved pain he is experiencing.

Before she met him, Grace was anxious and codependent. Tom has empowered her far more than her previous partners ever did. As she got to know him, she focused less on his diagnosis and more on him as a person. She says that she realizes he is not his BPD. They navigate his disorder together as just one thing that affects their relationship. She has become secure and strong and has grown a great deal personally since she met him. Learning how to set effective boundaries is key, and she has learned how to communicate with him more effectively.

She sometimes feels suffocated, but they discuss her feelings, and he goes to great lengths to ensure her happiness. She says that he has tremendous insight into what to do to ensure that their relationship works. Tom is loyal, devoted, and committed to the relationship.

Mark: Deciding to Make a Positive Split

When Mark first met Mandy, she was incredible—loving, patient, kind, understanding. She was everything he ever wanted in a woman, and the sex was great. He fell hard for her. After two and a half years, Mark proposed, and they married a year later.

It took about three months for him to see Mandy's violent rages. In retrospect, there were small red flags he'd missed. One night, when he couldn't sleep because she was snoring, he went to sleep in the spare room. In the morning, she told him their marriage was over. That was only the beginning. When he spent time with friends on the way home from a business trip, she accused him of cheating on her. She stopped wearing her wedding ring. She would swear at him when he tried to help her with everyday things like using the Wi-Fi. She abused him physically, telling him she wished he was dead. He took the blame for everything she said was wrong with their relationship and tried his best to fix things. Mandy kept breaking up with him then making up, sometimes several times a month. Eventually, Mark became suicidal and decided to move out temporarily and evaluate the situation. When he went home afterward, Mandy begged him to stay and, for the first and only time, opened up about her terrible childhood.

After Mark started therapy because of his suicidal feelings, his therapist gave him a book about BPD and got him to fill in a questionnaire—he answered all the questions positively. She then explained that Mandy suffered from BPD, and he wasn't the problem. He bought a copy of the book for his wife, and they attempted to work on things—Mandy wasn't too happy. They had one marriage counseling session, during which Mandy verbally love-bombed him in front of the therapist. Three weeks later, he went to the therapist alone, and she said she had seen right through Mandy's attempt to charm him and that it wasn't genuine. By then, Mark had left the relationship but still struggled with its intoxicating aftereffects. He isn't sure whether he will ever get over her completely.

Clare: An Exhausting Friendship

Clare's new friendship started off with a bang. Martha was great and funny, and it was easy to confide in her. The two got along well, but the friendship deepened quickly, which she realized afterward was a big red flag.

Martha gradually became more demanding. It was hard to pin down because she was very subtle and manipulative. She ignored Clare's boundaries and got angry whenever Clare told her no. Eventually, everything revolved around Martha and the chaos she created. There were always problems that only Clare could solve, and Martha needed constant validation and reassurance. Boundaries were crossed continuously because everything was an "emergency." She drew Clare away from her family, her life, and her work. However, because Clare felt Martha was a good friend, she wanted to help her. Eventually, Clare had to put her foot down—and that was when Martha revealed her true colors. She became nastier, and it was easier for Clare to see through her lies. She discovered Martha told tales about others constantly but was careful to insert some real facts to make it less obvious and make others feel sympathy for her. Clare eventually found the friendship exhausting and mentally draining. In between the episodes of neediness and manipulation, they had some great times together, and Clare would get sucked back in again.

Then something awful happened in Clare's life. Martha ignored Clare's distress and continued to pester Clare about helping her. She showed up unannounced at Clare's house, where Clare was crying over the tragedy that had occurred, and Clare was horrified to realize that Martha didn't even notice. Clare was devastated and realized that Martha didn't really care about her. Clare had been a great friend and given Martha everything she could, from reassurance and help to counseling and sympathizing. The day Clare experienced her own tragedy, she realized that everything she had given Martha wasn't enough. She always wanted more. Clare's needs weren't on Martha's radar. Clare found their friendship exhausting, confusing, and mentally draining. When she finally ended their friendship, she felt as though an enormous weight had been lifted. Martha has tried to get back into her life, but Clare is sticking to her decision.

Interactive Element: Putting Yourself First

If you feel that your relationship with your partner, friend, or coworker with BPD can no longer be maintained, it's time to plan your exit. Ask yourself the following questions to prepare for the breakup:

- What is your exit plan?
- Where can you go for support when you break up?
- Do you need somewhere else to stay, and who could assist you?
- How will you look after yourself mentally, emotionally, and physically after the breakup?
- How will you keep busy?

Key Takeaways

Breaking up is difficult—and can be even more challenging with a loved one with BPD, as they are more likely to react negatively. Consider talking things over with a counselor or your support group beforehand. Before proceeding, establish whether your partner intends to seek help (if they haven't) or go back to therapy and onto their medication if this has become erratic.

Leaving the relationship might be the only option if you're hopelessly overwhelmed, experiencing severe mental distress, being physically abused, witnessing self-harming behavior, or attempted suicide. Prepare and decide on your approach. Be calm and gentle but firm. Using DBT techniques can be helpful. Remember to validate them but stick to your decision.

After the breakup, allow yourself to experience your emotions. Develop an understanding of what happened and realize that everything was not your fault. It's preferable to cut communications, but if there are childcare issues involved, then keep contact to a minimum. Remove all online and offline tokens of the relationship. Surround yourself with positive, understanding people. Rekindle friendships, hobbies, and interests you might have neglected during your relationship. Talk to a counselor or therapist to disentangle yourself emotionally from your relationship. Practice self-care after the breakup to ensure your mental, emotional, and physical health and to facilitate healing.

Lighting the Road Ahead

There's no denying that there's still a lot of road ahead of you, but now that you have a deeper understanding of Borderline Personality Disorder and how to protect your own mental health at the same time as supporting your loved one, hopefully, it looks a little brighter. This is your chance to pass that hope on to someone else.

Simply by sharing your honest opinion of this book and a little about your own experience, you can help new readers find the guidance they so desperately need.

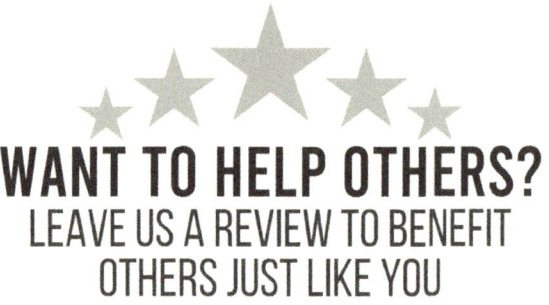

WANT TO HELP OTHERS?
LEAVE US A REVIEW TO BENEFIT OTHERS JUST LIKE YOU

Thank you so much for your support. You're making a huge difference.

Scan the QR code for a quick review!

Conclusion

Borderline Personality Disorder is a mental illness that affects a relatively small percentage of the North American population. However, its effects on relationships can be devastating for those with the diagnosis and their partners, spouses, family members, friends, or coworkers. BPD usually manifests when vulnerable individuals are in their late teens and early twenties. This relatively rare mental illness can be brought on by childhood neglect, as well as physical and sexual abuse. However, BPD might also have a biological root cause. In individuals with BPD, the parts of the brain that generate emotional responses are not effectively regulated by the more rational parts of the brain. This might explain BPD diagnoses where there is no family history of neglect or abuse.

Studies show that BPD may be inherited, with people more likely to develop the condition if close family members suffer from it. Women are more likely to be diagnosed with BPD; however, men are also affected. But are often misdiagnosed with other conditions, such as anger management issues or PTSD.

Symptoms often include intense emotional dysfunction with ecstatic highs and deep lows, black-and-white thinking, substance abuse, and dysfunctional relationships. Sufferers have a deep-seated fear of abandonment and a defective sense of self-worth.

In the initial stages of a relationship with a loved one with BPD, romantic partners and friends are drawn to the vivacious, attractive parts of their personas. Individuals with BPD mirror those around them, often becoming completely absorbed in their favorite person's interests or activities. This creates the illusion that they are highly compatible with potential romantic partners and friends. However, their fear of abandonment soon manifests, and they withdraw from the relationship to the consternation of the other people involved.

Individuals with BPD also exhibit recklessness, anger, rage, volatile emotional states, lying, and a lack of commitment. Dealing with these traits can be very stressful and frustrating for those in relationships with individuals with BPD. They rarely appreciate the achievements of others, the difficulties other people experience, or the efforts others make to appease them. Relationships can become one-sided, with the individual with BPD at the center and others supporting them.

Once someone is diagnosed with BPD, extensive therapy is usually required. Regular therapy is recommended but may prove ineffective. Interventions such as DBT, MBT, schema-focused therapy, STEPPS therapy, and transference-focused therapy can be very helpful and are often effective. Medication can also help to regulate anxiety, depression, and suicidal tendencies.

Support groups for sufferers, caregivers, family members, partners, and friends can help everyone navigate the complexities of the disorder. Caregivers for people with BPD need to look after their own physical health and mental well-being, as being close to an individual with BPD can be intense, demanding, stressful, and exhausting. Support groups are available for caregivers and families, and therapy might also be required.

Sometimes, someone in a relationship with a loved one with BPD may need to break off the relationship if it becomes too stressful, traumatic, or even dangerous. Breaking up should be handled carefully because of fear of abandonment, which may cause the BPD person to act in unpredictable ways. Using DBT techniques, remaining calm, and sticking to your decision are important when breaking up with a partner or friend with BPD. Surrounding yourself with supportive people, taking up hobbies and interests that make you happy, and finding someone to talk to about the emotions you may experience can all help with recovery.

When in treatment, the erratic behaviors of individuals with BPD can become regulated, and it is possible for them to form healthy and lasting relationships. These individuals are often intelligent, creative, emotionally intuitive, loyal, and committed once their BPD symptoms are under control. Those in positive relationships with people with BPD who are in treatment report having good relationships after learning to navigate the complexities of the disorder.

If you are in a relationship with someone with BPD, you know first-hand how difficult it is to withstand the emotional extremes they experience. As someone close to them, it's important for you to receive sufficient support, care for yourself, do things you enjoy, and consider therapy. It might also be important for you to know when to leave, should the nature of the relationship mean that this is an option for you.

Living with or having a relationship with someone who has BPD can be extremely challenging. I hope this book has helped you to better understand this personality disorder, as well as how to cope with the different aspects while maintaining your own mental and physical health.

References

5 ways to survive an argument with someone with BPD. (2019, August 2). Counselling Directory UK. https://www.counselling-directory.org.uk/memberarticles/5-ways-to-survive-an-argument-when-your-loved-one-has-borderline-personality-di

10 signs you're experiencing trauma after a toxic relationship. (2023, April 21). Counselling Directory UK. https://www.counselling-directory.org.uk/memberarticles/10-signs-youre-experiencing-trauma-after-a-toxic-relationship

ADAMHS. (2006, December 21). *Facts about borderline personality disorder (BPD) Board of Cuyahoga County.* https://www.adamhscc.org/resources/facts-about-mental-illness/borderline-personality-disorder#:~

Admin. (2020, February 4). *How to handle borderline personality disorder rage.* Clearview Treatment Programs. https://www.clearviewtreatment.com/resources/blog/how-to-handle-borderline-personality-disorder-rage/

Antonatos, L. (2022a, November 15). *12 things to know about dating someone with borderline personality disorder.* Choosing Therapy. https://www.choosingtherapy.com/dating-someone-with-bpd/

Antonatos, L. (2022b, December 2). *Borderline Rage: What It Is, Triggers & How to Manage.* Choosing Therapy. https://www.choosingtherapy.com/borderline-rage/

BPD Team. (2023, May 9). *The challenges of being in a relationship with someone with BPD.* BPD Borderline Personality Disorder. https://www.bpd.org.uk/in-a-relationship-with-someone-with-bpd/

Bennett, R. T. (n.d.). *A quote from The Light in the Heart.* Goodreads. https://www.goodreads.com/quotes/7553698-no-amount-of-regretting-can-change-the-past-and-no

Betterhelp Editorial Team. (2023, November 6). *Who is Marsha Linehan?* Betterhelp. https://www.betterhelp.com/advice/therapy/who-is-marsha-linehan/

Bozzatello, P., Rocca, P., Baldassdarri, L., Bosia, M., & Bellino, S. (2023). The role of trauma in early onset borderline personality disorder: A biopsychosocial perspective. *Frontiers in Psychiatry, 12.* https://doi.org/10.3389/fpsyt.2021.721361

BPD Family Communities. (2015, October 15). BPD Videos. https://www.bpdvideo.com/borderline-personality-disorder-online/communities/bpd-family

Brainy Quote. (n.d.-a). *If you are broken, you do not have to stay broken.* https://www.brainyquote.com/quotes/selena_gomez_802459?__cf_chl_tk=_aM4wCiGdzAbVqLUuS3uf7VlKGEya06VgoVKVJibRKE-1696923500-0-gaNycGzNFJA

Brainy Quote. (n.d.-b). *Looking forward quotes*. https://www.brainyquote.com/quotes/roy_cooper_1195062?src=t_looking_forward

Breaking up with someone who has borderline personality disorder. (2011, June 3). Borderline Personality Disorder Treatment. https://www.borderlinepersonalitytreatment.com/breaking-up-with-bpd.html

Carers, families, partners, and friends supporting people with borderline personality disorder. (2022, August 17). BPD Co. https://www.sahealth.sa.gov.au/wps/wcm/connect/public+content/sa+health+internet/services/mental+health+and+drug+and+alcohol+services/mental+health+services/borderline+personality+disorder+centre+of+excellence/supporting+people+with+borderline+personality+disorder/supporting+people+with+borderline+personality+disorder

Catchings, C. V. (2022, July 1). *Dating someone with BPD: What to expect*. Talkspace. https://www.talkspace.com/mental-health/conditions/borderline-personality-disorder/relationships-dating/

CDC. (2021, March 1). *Healthy eating tips*. Centers for Disease Control and Prevention. https://www.cdc.gov/nccdphp/dnpao/features/healthy-eating-tips/index.html

CDC. (2022, September 13). *Sleep hygiene tips — sleep and sleep disorders*. Centers for Disease Control and Prevention. https://www.cdc.gov/sleep/about_sleep/sleep_hygiene.html

Choi-kain, L. W., & Gunderson, J. G. (2009, July 31). *Borderline personality disorder and resistance to treatment*. Psychiatric Times. https://www.psychiatrictimes.com/view/borderline-personality-disorder-and-resistance-treatment

Christina. (2019). *Yes, it is possible!* Is it possible to recover from borderline personality disorder? https://www.quora.com/Why-would-a-diagnosed-BPD-refuse-therapy-What-are-they-afraid-of

Codependency and borderline personality disorder: How to spot it. (2012, June 7). Clearview Women's Center. https://www.borderlinepersonalitytreatment.com/codependency-and-borderline-personality-disorder-how-to-spot-it.html

Collins, H. (2023, March 20). *Brain biology, BPD & mindfulness*. New Harbinger Publications, Inc. https://www.newharbinger.com/blog/professional/brain-biology-bpd-mindfulness/

Crumpler, C. (2022, May 27). *Mindfulness for beginners: How to get started*. Psych Central. https://psychcentral.com/health/new-to-mindfulness-how-to-get-started#how-to-practice

Davila, J. (2016, June 17). *Stop trying to fix things; just listen!* Psychology Today United Kingdom. https://www.psychologytoday.com/gb/blog/skills-healthy-relationships/201606/stop-trying-fix-things-just-listen

Dodgson, L. (2023, May 10). *These are the 3 types of attachment styles — and how each affects your relationships*. Business Insider. https://www.insider.com/the-3-different-attachment-styles-2018-6

Eagle, R. (2020, November 18). *Five therapies for borderline personality disorder (BPD)*. Medical News Today. https://www.medicalnewstoday.com/articles/therapies-for-bpd#is-it-a-cure

Eightify. (2023, September 30). *Essential post-breakup insights for BPD relationships*. https://eightify.app/summary/relationships/essential-post-breakup-insights-for-bpd-relationships

Galen, G. (2016). Validation: Making sense of the emotional turmoil in borderline personality disorder. McLean Hospital. https://www.mcleanhospital.org/sites/default/files/shared/BPDWebinar-Galen-Validation-Webinar10.13.16.pdf

Giffin, J. (2008, September). *Family experience of borderline personality disorder*. Anzift, 133–138. https://bpdfoundation.org.au/images/Jan_Giffin_Family%20expe rience%20of%20BPD.pdf

Gilette, H. (2021, December 14). *How do people with borderline personality disorder act in relationships?* Psych Central. https://psychcentral.com/disorders/borderline-personality-relationships-cycle

Gillihan, S. J. (2023, April 4). *12 signs a past trauma may be affecting your relationship*. Psychology Today United Kingdom. https://www.psychologytoday.com/gb/blog/think-act-be/202304/12-signs-a-past-trauma-may-be-affecting-your-relationship

Gordon, S. (2023, December 4). *How to find connection when you really need it*. Verywell Mind. https://www.verywellmind.com/what-to-do-when-you-need-someone-to-talk-to-5089236

Gould, W. R. (2022, November 7). *What is codependency?* Verywell Mind. https://www.verywellmind.com/what-is-codependency-5072124#:~

Green, J. (n.d.). *A quote from Turtles All the Way Down*. GoodReads. https://www.goodreads.com/quotes/8848435-there-is-hope-even-when-your-brain-tells-you-there

Grouport. (n.d.). *Supporting a partner with borderline personality disorder: Tips for navigating the emotional landscape*. Grouport Journal. https://www.grouporttherapy.com/blog/bpd-partners#:~

Helping a loved one with BPD: 6 ways to stop enabling their behaviors. (2011, November 16). Clearview Women's Center. https://www.borderlinepersonalitytreatment.com/preventing-enabling-behavior.html

How to set boundaries and say no to someone with BPD. (2023, February 27). Veritas Psychotherapy. https://veritaspsychotherapy.ca/blog/saying-no-to-someone-with-bpd/

Humphries, T. (2020, March 13). *Hold space, not ropes: The difference between compassion and codependency*. Sober Recovery. https://www.soberrecovery.com/recovery/hold-space-not-ropes/

"I" statements instead of "you" statements in arguments. (2022, November 8). Relationships Australia. https://www.relationshipsnsw.org.au/blog/i-statements-vs-you-statements/

Johnson, R. S. (2020a, July 20). *Surviving a breakup when your partner has borderline personality disorder.* BDP Family. https://www.bpdfamily.com/content/surviving-break-when-your-partner-has-borderline-personality

Johnson, R. S. (2020b, August 13). *Anosognosia and getting a "borderline" into therapy.* BPD Family. https://www.bpdfamily.com/content/how-to-get-borderline-into-therapy

Johnston, E. (2022, March 16). *How using "I feel" statements can help you communicate.* Verywell Mind. https://www.verywellmind.com/what-are-feeling-statements-425163

Jones, M. (2023). *How to encourage someone to see a therapist.* NAMI. https://www.nami.org/Blogs/NAMI-Blog/November-2017/How-to-Encourage-Someone-to-See-a-Therapist?utm_source=naminow&utm_medium=email&utm_campaign=naminow

Josifovska, M. (2023, May 17). *Famous people & celebrities with BPD (borderline personality disorder).* Screen and Reveal. https://screenandreveal.com/celebrities-with-bpd/

Kay, M. L., Poggenpoel, M., Myburgh, C. P., & Downing, C. (2018). *Experiences of family members who have a relative diagnosed with borderline personality disorder.* Curationis, *41*(1). https://doi.org/10.4102/curationis.v41i1.1892

Keen, G. (2022, June 5). *How to forget BPD ex?* BPD Aid. https://bpdaid.com/how-to-forget-bpd-ex/

Kreisman, J. (2018, November 7). *Confronting conflict in borderline personality disorder.* Psychology Today United Kingdom. https://www.psychologytoday.com/gb/blog/i-hate-you-dont-leave-me/201810/confronting-conflict-in-borderline-personality-disorder

Kristi. (2020, January 9). *Causes of borderline personality disorder.* Bridges to Recovery. https://www.bridgestorecovery.com/borderline-personality-disorder/causes-of-borderline-personality-disorder/

Krouse, L. (2023, November 29). *How to receive a borderline personality disorder diagnosis.* Verywell Health. https://www.verywellhealth.com/borderline-personality-disorder-diagnosis-5101625#:~

Krstic, Z., & Dolgoff, S. (2022, November 9). *Change your life in 45 days thanks to these simple self-care tasks.* Good Housekeeping. https://www.goodhousekeeping.com/health/wellness/g25643343/self-care-ideas/

Lawrenz, L. (2023, November 20). *Why you may experience emotional detachment and what to do about it.* Healthline. https://www.healthline.com/health/mental-health/emotional-detachment#treatment

Leary, M. (2017). *How can people with borderline personality disorder recover?* Quora. https://www.quora.com/Why-would-a-diagnosed-BPD-refuse-therapy-What-are-they-afraid-of

Leaving a relationship with someone with borderline personality disorder. Grouport Journal.

(n.d.). https://www.grouporttherapy.com/blog/leaving-someone-with-border
line-personality-disorder

Lee, C. I. (2022, July 12). *Setting boundaries without guilt — is it possible?* LA Concierge
Psychologist. https://laconciergepsychologist.com/blog/setting-boundaries-
without-guilt/#:~:

Les Miserables. (n.d.). *A quote from Les Misérables.* GoodReads. https://www.
goodreads.com/quotes/10095-even-the-darkest-night-will-end-and-the-sun-
will

Lo, I. (2022, August 12). *The potential upsides to having a partner with borderline.*
Psychology Today United Kingdom. https://www.psychologytoday.com/gb/
blog/living-emotional-intensity/202208/the-potential-upsides-having-partner-
borderline

Lobel, D. S. (2020, December 22). *Enabling borderline personality disorder.* Psychology
Today United Kingdom. https://www.psychologytoday.com/gb/blog/my-
side-the-couch/202012/enabling-borderline-personality-disorder

Lobel, D. S. (2021, September 22). *How borderline personality disorder can tear families
apart.* Psychology Today South Africa. https://www.psychologytoday.com/za/
blog/my-side-the-couch/202109/how-borderline-personality-disorder-can-
tear-families-apart

Majsiak, B., & Young, C. (2022, June 3). *5 ways to practice breath-focused meditation,*
Everyday Health. https://www.everydayhealth.com/alternative-health/living-
with/ways-practice-breath-focused-meditation/

Marley, B. (n.d.). *Bob Marley quote: "You never know how strong you are, until being strong is
your only choice."* Quotefancy.com. https://quotefancy.com/quote/35454/Bob-
Marley-You-never-know-how-strong-you-are-until-being-strong-is-your-only-
choice

Martin, S. (2020, April 23). *7 types of boundaries you may need.* Psych Central. https://
psychcentral.com/blog/imperfect/2020/04/7-types-of-boundaries-you-may-
need

Mayo, G. (2023). *Been with my BPD partner for a year.* Can Anyone Give Success
Stories on How They Overcame a BPD Relationship? https://www.quora.
com/We-hear-too-much-about-how-painful-BPD-relationships-are-Can-
anyone-give-success-stories-on-how-they-overcame-a-BPD-relationship

Mental Health Foundation. (2022). *How to look after your mental health using exercise.*
Mental Health Foundation. https://www.mentalhealth.org.uk/explore-mental-
health/publications/how-look-after-your-mental-health-using-exercise

Migala, J. (2022, October 25). *Is borderline personality disorder genetic?* EverydayHealth.
https://www.everydayhealth.com/bpd/borderline-personality-disorder-are-
your-genes-blame/#:~

Mind. (2022, September). *Borderline personality disorder (BPD) — how can other people
help?* Mind. https://www.mind.org.uk/information-support/types-of-mental-

health-problems/borderline-personality-disorder-bpd/for-friends-and-family/ #LearnMoreAboutBPD

Montemurro, F. (2011). *"I" messages or "I" statements*. BUMC. https://www.bumc. bu.edu/facdev-medicine/files/2011/08/I-messages-handout.pdf

Moore, M. (2022, September 8). *Here's 3 ways boundaries can help you*. Psych Central. https://psychcentral.com/relationships/the-importance-of-personal-bound aries#What-is-a-boundary

NIMH. (2022). *Caring for your mental health*. National Institute of Mental Health. https://www.nimh.nih.gov/health/topics/caring-for-your-mental-health#:~

NIMH. (2023, April). *Borderline personality disorder*. National Institute for Mental Health. https://www.nimh.nih.gov/health/topics/borderline-personality- disorder

NEABPD. (2011, July 8). *The family connections program*. National Education Alliance for Borderline Personality Disorder. https://www.borderlinepersonalitydisor der.org/family-connections/

O'Dougherty, M. (2021, November 22). *The benefit of support groups when you love someone with borderline personality disorder*. National Alliance on Mental Illness. https://www.nami.org/Blogs/NAMI-Blog/November-2021/The-Benefit-of- Support-Groups-When-You-Love-Someone-with-Borderline-Personality- Disorder

Oberg, B. (2012, March 20). *Does borderline personality disorder make you codependent?* HealthyPlace. https://www.healthyplace.com/blogs/borderline/2012/03/the- family-secret-bpd-and-codependency

Pattemore, C. (2021, April 19). *Borderline personality disorder: Myths vs. facts*. Psych Central. https://psychcentral.com/blog/borderline-personality-disorder-facts- vs-myths#fact-vs-fiction

Perry, E. (2021, August 23). *Seeking help for your mental health is brave. And beneficial*. BetterUp. https://www.betterup.com/blog/seeking-help

Physiopedia. (n.d.). *Limbic system*. https://www.physio-pedia.com/Limbic_Sys tem#:~

Porr, V. (2019). *A family guide to validation*. Asmile. https://asmile.org.au/wp- content/uploads/2019/06/BPD_familyGuide.pdf

Quora. (2023, September). *What is it like to be in a relationship with someone with border- line personality disorder, (aka emotionally unstable personality disorder...* Quora. https:// www.quora.com/What-is-it-like-to-be-in-a-relationship-with-someone-with- borderline-personality-disorder-aka-emotionally-unstable-personality-disorder- and-emotional-dysregulation-disorder

Responding to challenging behavior. (2018, July 19). Borderline in the ACT. https:// www.borderlineintheact.org.au/service-providers-working-with-people-with- bpd/responding-to-challenging-behaviour/

Revelant, J. (2018, October 15). *Tips for couples living with borderline personality disorder*.

Everyday Health. https://www.everydayhealth.com/bpd/tips-couples-living-with-borderline-personality-disorder/#:~

Rice, M. (2023, January 23). *How to stop being codependent: 9 helpful tips.* Talkspace. https://www.talkspace.com/blog/how-to-stop-being-codependent/

Robb-Dover, K. (2022, April 16). *When to leave someone with BPD (borderline personality disorder).* FHE Health. https://fherehab.com/learning/when-to-leave-some one-with-bpd#:~

Rope, K. (2021, April 26). *How to handle a relationship with someone who has borderline personality disorder.* WebMD. https://www.webmd.com/mental-health/features/borderline-personality-disorder-relationship

Salter-Pednault, K. (2020, February 10). *Borderline personality disorder treatment.* Verywell Mind. https://www.verywellmind.com/borderline-personality-disorder-treatment-425451

Salters-Pednault, K. (2022, December 5). *Healthy coping skills for people with borderline personality disorder.* Verywell Mind. https://www.verywellmind.com/coping-skills-borderline-personality-disorder-425412

Salters-Pednault, K. (2020, November 25). *Striking statistics about borderline personality disorder in the U.S.* Verywell Mind. https://www.verywellmind.com/borderline-personality-disorder-statistics-425481#:~

Sansone, R. A., & Sansone, L. A. (2012). *Employment in borderline personality disorder.* Innovations in Clinical Neuroscience, *9*(9), 25–29. https://www.ncbi.nlm.nih.gov/pmc/articles/PMC3472897/#:~:

Smith, C. (2019). *What is a borderline like as a friend?* Quora. https://www.quora.com/What-is-it-like-to-have-a-close-friend-with-borderline-PD

Smith, M. (2019). *Helping someone with borderline personality disorder.* HelpGuide. https://www.helpguide.org/articles/mental-disorders/helping-someone-with-borderline-personality-disorder.htm

Spelman, D. B. (2022, June 14). *7 stages of a BPD relationship.* Private Therapy Clinic. https://theprivatetherapyclinic.co.uk/blog/7-stages-of-a-bpd-relationship/

Steber, C. (2021, May 20). *10 signs you're experiencing trauma after a toxic relationship.* Counselling Directory UK. https://www.counselling-directory.org.uk/member articles/10-signs-youre-experiencing-trauma-after-a-toxic-relationship

Taylor, M. (2019). *What is it like dating someone with borderline personality disorder?* What Are Some Real-Life Stories of Those Involved in Any Kind of Relationship with Borderline Personality Disorder? https://www.quora.com/What-are-some-real-life-stories-of-those-involved-in-any-kind-of-relationship-with-border line-personality-disorder-sufferers

Terrighena, E. (2022, November 2). *Borderline personality disorder busting myths.* Mind-Balance. https://www.mind-balance.org/post/borderline-personality-disorder-busting-myths#:~

Thowfeek, T. (n.d.). *Boundaries*. Out of the FOG. https://outofthefog.website/what-to-do-2/2015/12/3/boundaries

United For Now. (2009, May 19). *1.22 | Are you supporting or enabling?* BPD Family. https://bpdfamily.com/message_board/index.php?topic=95263.0

What is it like to have a close friend with borderline PD? (n.d.). Quora. https://www.quora.com/What-is-it-like-to-have-a-close-friend-with-borderline-PD

Why is setting boundaries with a person with borderline personality disorder (BPD) so difficult? (n.d.). My Side of the Couch. https://www.mysideofthecouch.com/blogs/why-is-setting-boundaries-with-a-person-with-borderline-personality-disorder-bpd-so-difficult

Why would a diagnosed BPD refuse therapy? What are they afraid of? (n.d.). Quora. https://www.quora.com/Why-would-a-diagnosed-BPD-refuse-therapy-What-are-they-afraid-of

Wilson, J. (2022, November 23). *What to do if you feel guilty after setting boundaries*. HuffPost UK. https://www.huffingtonpost.co.uk/entry/setting-boundaries-without-guilt_l_637b8f09e4b0c5739622d69f

Zambon, V. (2020, November 6). *How can borderline personality disorder affect relationships?* Medical News Today. https://www.medicalnewstoday.com/articles/borderline-personality-disorder-relationships#effects-on-relationships

Made in the USA
Las Vegas, NV
16 October 2024

97017336R00094